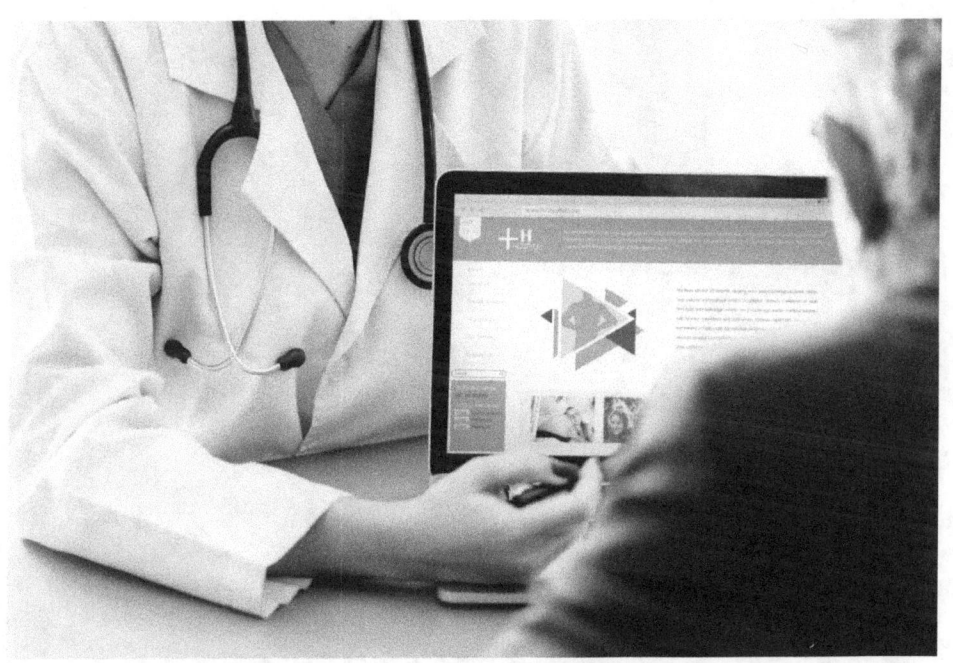

Healthcare Decoded

By

Harish C. Rijhwani

© copyright 2019 Harish Rijhwani

Foreword

I have always known of Harish as someone who wants to understand the 'why' of things, get to the bottom of everything. As a child, I saw him dismantle expensive shiny toys like cars and engines that would have been just gifted to him. He would dismantle a toy car, for instance; part by part, spend hours at it and then spend another few precious hours rebuilding the piece. That is what this book is about in a way.

Harish breaks down the subject bit by bit and simplifies what to some people, maybe rocket science: IT in healthcare. His personal anecdotes and conversational style make it an easy, delightful read. 'Healthcare Decoded,' true to its name takes us through the journey of how healthcare was practiced in early days, the health care practice today with details on insurance, data collection and the probable future of healthcare with devices in patient's hands. This book is for someone who wants to understand the history, the present, and the possible future of IT in healthcare and enjoy the journey along the way.

Heena Kanal is a communications professional with 25 years of experience in industries such as IT, FMCG, lifestyle, and healthcare. Currently, she leads communications globally for a leading pharma company. Views are personal.

Preface

The basis of this book stems from my desire to learn and explore the IT side of Healthcare. I wanted a means to share my knowledge with my students, as well as my colleagues. I have tried to express my knowledge in a simple and fun way where even a Non-Healthcare/Non-IT person could understand the same. Many of the examples shared in the book are my own, and I have tried to relate the same. There are many more concepts which I would like to add in the future, though some of these concepts could be more technical but very much around healthcare.

In truth, I would not have reached where I have without a strong support group. Primarily my family (my mother, sister, and wife) and my colleagues and mentors who have supported me all the way. Thank you all for your unwavering support.

Table of Contents

#1: Mr. Shingles & Mr. Future Pox

It is a cold Thursday morning in Nashville though it's February (the year is 2006). It is almost the end of my business trip only three weeks before I leave for India Yippee! I am staying at Ridgelake, a very beautiful place; there are quite a lot of amenities within the area. A swimming pool, squash court, tennis court, the only thing missing was a cricket pitch ☺.

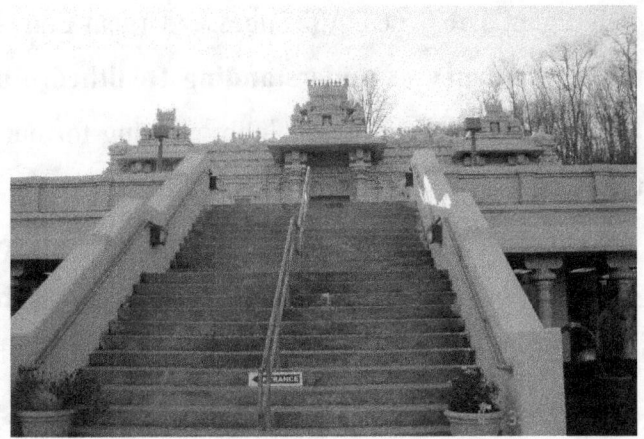

There even was a temple nearby known as the Ganesh Temple. My colleague, who stayed nearby, was recently diagnosed with Shingles (a painful rash, which is a reactivation of the chicken pox virus). Though he was supposed to stay at home, he decided to come to the office. Well, unfortunately, he was told to Go Back Home and not show so much dedication towards work. Here is where things started to change cause just a couple of days before we were playing Squash!!

On that morning, I noticed my body had small red spots coming up, even on my head, I could feel small bumps coming up. I ignored the same and went to the office. In the night I decided to use some telemedicine and took a photograph and emailed the same to my Aunt in Washington, who is a radiologist. At that time, WhatsApp did not exist, so we had to use this primitive method of communicating☺. After sending the photo, I called and asked her, but as the photo was not so great, we could conclude that it was a simple rash.

The next day morning the spots seemed bigger, so my colleague with whom I was staying with (not Mr. Shingles, Mr. Future Pox) decided to take me to an urgent care – TUCA (Tennessee Urgent Care Associates). **{This is where my journey of understanding Healthcare began}**. We reached TUCA and went and sat in the lobby waiting for our turn. Till I waited my turn came, I was handed a form to fill up which had all the information around my name, age, gender, and other information related to my Insurance. Since I was on a business trip, I had insurance, but I did not have an insurance card. So, what did that imply? Well, I had to pay from my pocket and get the same reimbursed directly from the Insurance company. We waited 20-30 minutes in the lobby before my turn came. Once my turn came, we went to the examination room where the nurse came and asked me some more questions. The nurse also had a form with her clipped on a writing pad. She asked me various questions around my lifestyle for example –

- Do you Smoke?

- Do you Drink?
- Are you on any medication?

Along with this, she also took my vitals in terms of Blood pressure, height, weight, and temperature. All this information she noted down on the form. After all of this is when arrived the hero of the movie – "The Physician," The physician looked at the information filled on the chart by the nurse, then looked at the spots and said – Ok So you have Chicken Pox...

Oh, My God!! Here I was making plans to go back, and now I would not be able to travel since I had the Pox (contagious you know – like Shingles). It is important to note that the Chicken Pox Virus causes Shingles. The other reason why it was important for me to reach home as I had an interview for my Part-Time MBA around 17th Feb, and here I was around three weeks from that date unable to travel.

The Physician then gave me my prescription and gave me a date for my next visit, which was around 7-8 days away. It was now time to leave, and I had to pay a bill of approx. $200/- out of my pocket, note that this did not include the bill for medications which I had to buy from a nearby pharmacy. After the visit, Mr. Future Pox and I went to the nearby pharmacy to buy my medications. It was interesting to note that the medications provided to me were in custom boxes, i.e., the box had the medication name as well as my name (Patient's name). I found this new, as this is not how I bought medications in India.

The next time when I went for a follow up (after around four days I think so) I did not have to wait, I was told to go and directly sit in the room (this was because I had Chicken Pox – contagious you know!!). Then I went for one final time where the Physician even gave me a certificate stating I can travel. So, I packed my bags reached India on 18th Feb, gave my interview on the last day of the schedule, which was 19th Feb. Luckily, I did well and went on to do my Part-Time MBA for three years – evening (6:45 pm to 9:15 pm) and weekend classes.

By the way, you might be wondering why am I calling Mr. Future Pox as Mr. Future Pox. The reason being he returned to India after four weeks from the date of my departure. Unluckily he got the Pox on the plane while returning to India! ☺

#2 Chronology of Healthcare

Healthcare is a highly Complex Industry. Even as a patient if one has a health problem, one wonders who I should visit. I should go to the Emergency/Casualty/Urgent care or my General Physician or a specialist. Highly confusing and at times, even frustrating!!!

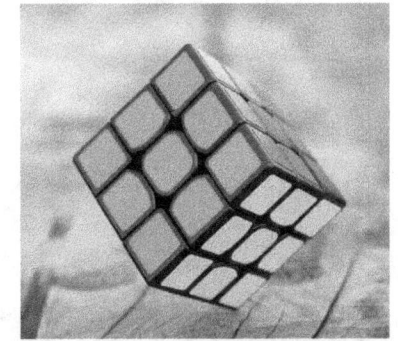

But things don't stop here; finding the right Physician is just the beginning. The fun part begins right after/during your visit because this is when all other healthcare entities (Insurance Companies, Pharmaceuticals, Medical Devices, and many others) become part of the movie scene.

In order to decode the confusing Maze of Healthcare, we need first to enter the same, and the only way to do so is to start with the Basics. You know when I was doing my MBA, we had a subject "Integrated Marketing," and we were discussing the Primary purpose of a Phone. If I go back to the '90s when we did not have mobiles/cell phones, the only reason why a phone existed was to communicate with others. In simple words make a phone call, everything else additional we get now is an Add-On. Similar lines, if I ask the question, what is the primary purpose/goal of Healthcare? The answer should be pretty straight forward – "To Provide Care."

At one point or the other, we have all visited a Physician, and to a certain extent, are aware of how one receives Care nowadays. But do you know how one received care earlier?

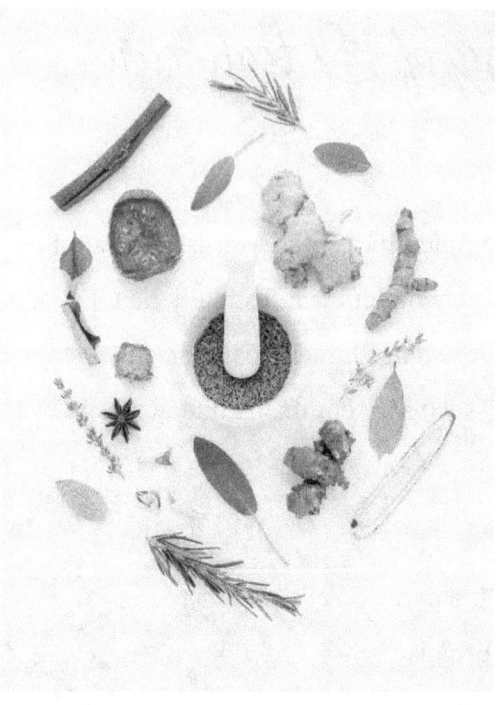

In India, we know herbs were used to treat patients, i.e., Ayurveda. If we look at history specifically in ancient times, the health of an individual was managed within the home of an individual – a.k.a. Home Remedies. Treatment was done using herbs – flora, and fauna during these times. This knowledge was passed from one generation to another, but at that time, people still did not understand the underlying reason why a specific sickness was happening. Many cultures started to study this subject then, and people started to document medicine.

The earliest reference of documented medicine is from Mesopotamian (somewhere between current Iran and Kuwait). These Tablets were in use around 1600 BC, and quite a few are present in the British Museum. In Ancient times people who were experts in herbs and medicines existed and were called as "physicians."

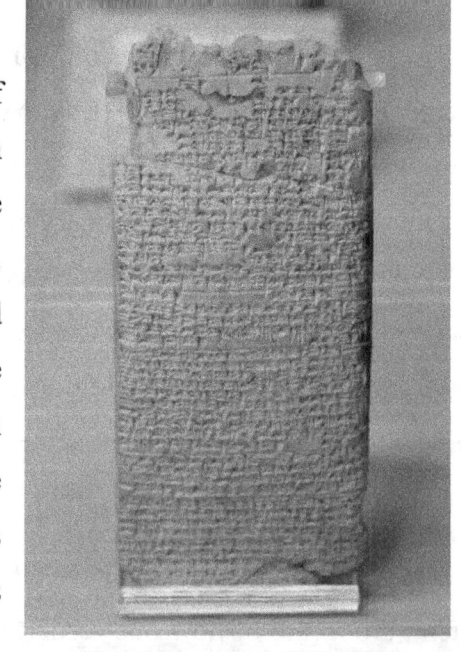

Figure: Sumerian medical tablet

So, when exactly did the world see a change in how we treat patients, Any Thoughts?? Ok if you are scratching your head and thinking Darwin's Theory, Maslow's law then that's not it ☺.

In the 19th and 20th centuries, quite a few technological advances happened in the world, and all focused towards research on specific diseases (Therapeutic Revolution). Diseases were linked to microorganisms (Germ Theory) and vaccines started to get developed for the same. There was a growth seen in biomedicine and along with this came globalization of medicine. In this era, we also saw many new devices such as X-rays, antiseptics, and newer means of diagnosing a patient's problem. If we look at the time frame, this was also the time Britain was colonizing the world, and due to this, there was a rise in Infectious Diseases. The 1920 Influenza virus infected over 500 million people around the world and killed around 100 million. Overall there was an increased focus on public health and investing in surveillance systems. There was also a focus on eradicating specific diseases such as smallpox - this approach was called a Vertical health approach (Top Down). This Approach faced a lot of criticism as using this method did not result in the eradication of other diseases. It is at this juncture around the 1970s realization struck that improving medical care cannot be the only aspect used to improve health and social conditions.

We need other entities/sectors also to get involved; this fueled the need for building basic Health Services (Bottom Up). Hopefully, the above 600 words / 3000 characters were interesting, and we also spoke about quite a few entities which we need to understand as part of our basics.

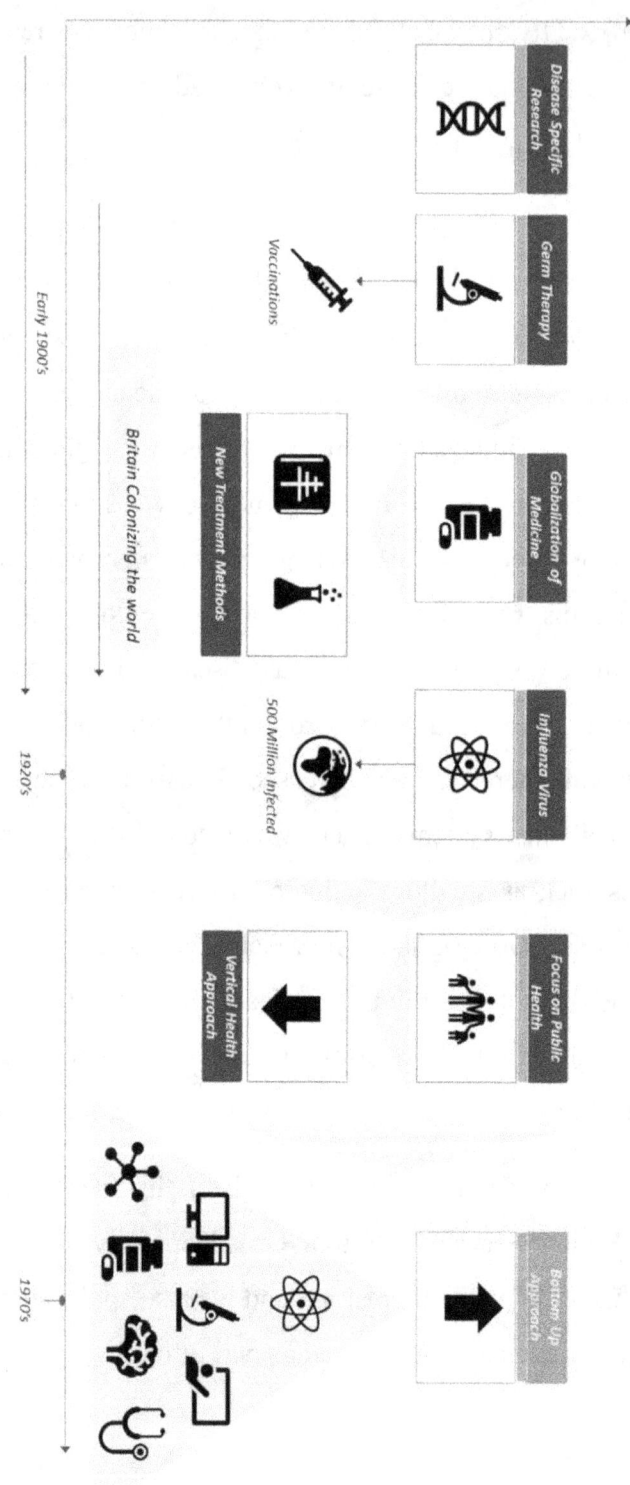

Let us quickly look at these entities.

1. The key entity here is the **Patient** – the person who needs care.

2. A **Physician/Healer** – The person who provides care to the Patient

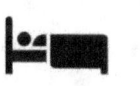 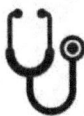  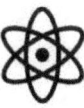 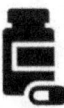

3. **Governments** – primary responsibility was improving Public Health and creating the infrastructure for providing basic Health Services.

Now were there more, oh yeah there were

4. **Research Organizations** – These are life science organizations (LS) focused on studying micro-organisms (remember Germ Therapy).

5. **Medical Devices** – These Organizations create new devices for improved treatments of patients.

6. **Pharmaceuticals** – We talked about creating vaccines; this is done by Pharma companies who focus on developing new medicines for the treatment of diseases.

You might be aware in Each industry there is always a First Mover Advantage, on similar lines do you know which was the 1st Hospital? I know that Wisselbank was one of the 1st Banks to be established in 1609. I was not able to exactly find out the name of a specific Hospital which got established first, but it is interesting to know that "Early 200 to 400 BC have documented the use of temples and institutions to treat patients in Greece, Rome, and India". That is correct ancient Greece had temples of Asclepius (The Greek God of Medicine & healing), which was later adopted by Romans. In India, cities had built houses for dispensing charity and medicine. These are some of the examples of the earliest documentary evidence where institutes provided care to the sick.

By the way, if you can find out which was the 1st Hospital established do let me know ☺

#3 The Rise of Health Insurance

We know that 200 years back Hospitals existed, but patients were mostly given treatment at their homes in most cases, even childbirth happened at home. But now there are Hospitals and also a Healthcare Insurance company; and along with them you have a claim form (A UB04, CMS1500 or a Superbill). To understand how this Healthcare Industry reached the current stage, we need to deep dive into some history, and you might find this very interesting, so read on.

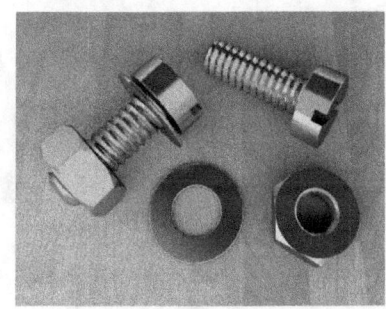

To understand the current some aspects of Health Insurance, we need to go back in Time to around 1800s. Around 1801 Eli Whitney demonstrated the concept of "Interchangeable Parts" specifically for Firearms. You might be wondering what Interchangeable is? Well, in simple words, they are components (Example: nuts & bolts) which are identical to each other and can replace another similar part.

The 1800s was the time when coal power and machine production were changing the world. Peter Cooper in 1830 designed and developed the 1st Steam powered Locomotive (called as Tom Thumb) in the US and 1850 we saw a rise of the Manufacturing Industry, mass production of goods (using

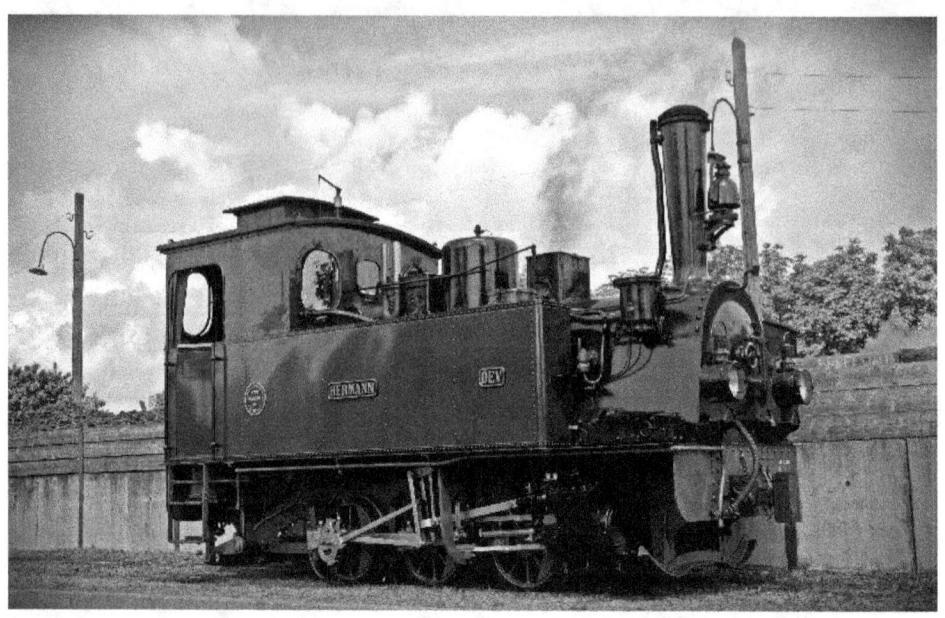

the concept of Interchangeable Parts). So where is the link with Healthcare here?

Well, it is interesting to note that one of the 1st Health Assurance's was for Accidents which could happen while building railroads and steamboats and this was provided by "Franklin Health Assurance Company of Massachusetts."

It is also important to note that at this point Physicians did not have a fixed fee; in most parts of the world, an *"honorarium,"* was given, which is more like a thank you gift. For all you know they might have also got grains and pulses for their services ☺. The situation in the US was slightly different as here you 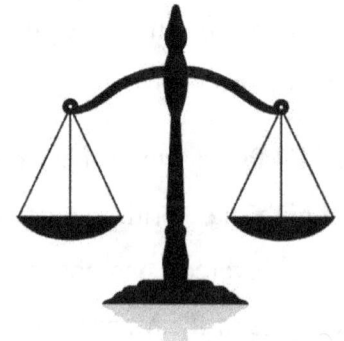 could buy Drugs/Medical services as you would buy something from a grocer's store. In some cases, the Physicians would charge you based on what you could afford. If you were rich, you were charged more; if you were poor, the cost of treatment would be less. This concept was known as Sliding scale.

Some might argue that this method was correct, and some might say this is incorrect. The Physician's argued by this method that, they were providing healthcare to all patients rich and poor equally. But when you compare this situation currently, it is the opposite (The scale has turned), and people having health insurance pay less while those who do not will pay more.

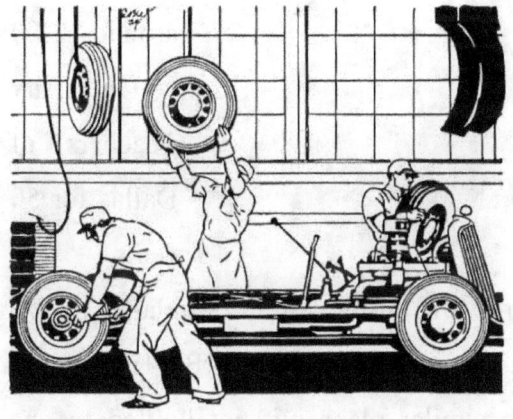

The advent of the 19th Century saw the Industrial Revolution and the 1st Moving Assembly line (Ford in 1913) and the people working on shop floors. Accidents were common in organizations on the shop floor, and employers were liable for injuries due to negligence. To defend such cases organization argued in multiple ways one being the risk was part of the contract other it was the workers' fault. One reform which came between 1910 to 1915 (enacted by 32 states) was "Workers Compensation" where employers could buy insurance coverage by their state. An interesting change at this point was that employers started to hire physicians to provide care, and due to this, there was a decline in the volume of work for local physicians.

The end of 1929 saw the beginning of "The Great Depression" causing a reduction in demand for goods and services worldwide and affected Local Hospitals, causing occupancy rates to drop and charity to increase. Patients were unable to pay their hospital bills, and hospitals needed money, one such Hospital was Baylor University Hospital. To come out of this situation, Justin Ford Kimble (Administrator at Baylor hospital) 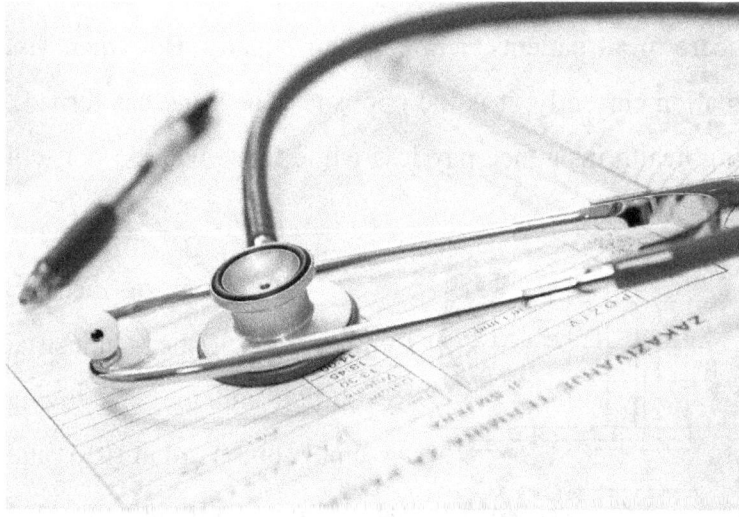 offered a plan for providing 21 days Hospital Services to around 1200 University Teachers of Dallas for 50 cents per month. This plan was limited to only one hospital and is similar to a PPO (Preferred Provider Organization) Plan in current times. By 1932, other hospitals started coming out with similar plans but not limited to one hospital. Hospitals started working with the American Health Association (AHA) to approve Hospital Approved Plans. In 1946, this came to be known as the Blue Cross Commission.

States did not view this concept as Insurance, but an advance payment of services (Like a Prepaid Card). The New York State commissioner in 1933 ruled that this needs to be viewed as "Insurance" because the hospital is taking an advance to provide services in the future. So, what 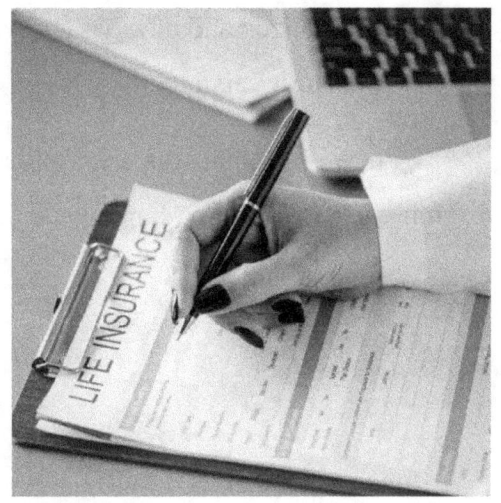 does this imply? Simply that the plans need to start complying with Insurance Laws. After this, in 1939 came Blue Shield, which was similar to Blue Cross only difference being it was to provide Insurance for Physician Services.

After World War II in 1945, there was a focus on creating a National Health Insurance Plan (Medicare and Medicaid), and in 1964 we saw the enactment of Health Insurance for the elderly known as Medicare in current times. This Medicare Plan has over the years evolved in 4 parts, Medicare Part A (Inpatient), Part B(Preventive), Part C (Medicare Advantage: A + B & vision, dental) and Part D (Prescription Drugs).

In parallel, there was also a focus to standardize the billing process and to use one single form for reimbursement. Thirteen different forms were developed Jointly by AHA and HFMA (Healthcare Financial Management Association) and rejected between the years 1968 to 1972. The 14th version of the form (UB-16-78) was developed, updated field tested in Georgia and later piloted in 5 states. In 1975 NUBC (National Uniform Billing Committee) was formed to maintain and develop this form. Finally, in 1982,

UB-82 was finalized and now has evolved from UB-82 to UB-92 to UB-04, which is the latest version.

Phew, now that was a long journey to start around the 1800s and reach to the current point, hope you enjoyed the journey!

#4 Managing the Revenue

During my MBA, we were asked to read the book "The Goal" by Eliyahu Goldratt. The book talks about various aspects of continuous improvements and the theory of constraints. One of the points which I always remember from the book is the Question asked, "What is the Goal of a Company?"

"The Goal of any company is to make money," this holds for all companies considering they are for-profit. Hence, it is very important we understand the Billing process in a hospital in a bit more detail, though we did cover the same briefly as part of the preface. Whenever I try to explain this in class, I try to use roleplay as it is fun, but let's see if I can write it in the same way.

Nobody likes going to a hospital believe me; it is not like visiting an ATM

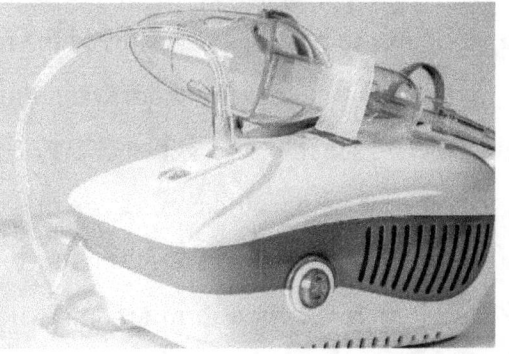

to withdraw money. So, when my mother was not feeling well, we first called the Physician for a home visit. She was having some breathing problems, and the Physician gave some medications –Antibiotic and Montec AB for possibly Bronchospasm. She felt a little better after some time but was still having some trouble breathing. So, I spoke with the Physician the next day at 7:30 AM, and he said do Nebulization and get a chest X-Ray done.

"Nebulization," that's the first time I heard that word and when I googled the same I read the below from Wikipedia, "*In medicine, a nebulizer or nebulizer is a drug delivery device used to administer medication in the form of a mist inhaled into the lungs*." So basically, one can't just take some medication off the shelf and pop it like a pill. I went to my local chemist and asked him I need to do nebulization. He showed me the machine of MEDTECH – Handyneb Smart. He opened the same and explained to me some of the things like "This is the mask," "you connect this pipe here" and "you put the medicine here." Medicine?? Medicine??, I thought, what medicine do I use? the Physician did not tell me any medicine.

I tried calling him and but was unable to reach him. Finally, I asked the pharmacist what we can use? He said for the time being use "Sterile water," which is safe and will give some relief until you can connect with the Physician. So, I bought the machine and some sterile water (they looked like small plastic injections). My mom did the nebulization and got some relief, in the meantime I was able to connect with the Physician, and the Physician said use Duolin respules and one more medicine whose name I am unable to recall. So that solved the nebulization puzzle, but we still had to do an X-Ray, but my mom was in no condition to move around, so we decided to see if we can get an X-Ray done at home. The Physician referred to someone who would come to do the X-Ray with a portable machine. The person came home in the afternoon to do the X-ray but while doing so caused more exertion to my mom. Before the X-ray technician came, she was feeling stable, but after the X-ray, she wasn't feeling great and was having trouble breathing.

We tried everything we could from the "Homecare" perspective, and there wasn't any option left but to go to the hospital. At around 5.30/6.00 pm, my sister called for an Ambulance, and we took my mom to the nearest hospital. Once we reached there, we took my Mom to the casualty ward. As soon as we entered, two nurses moved her to a casualty bed, and the Physician converged towards her to 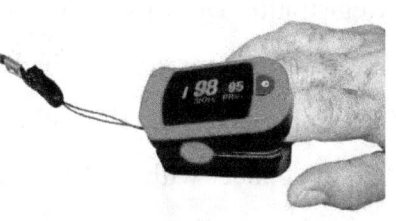 understand what happened. One nurse was checking her vitals – Blood pressure, another nurse connected some device on her finger, which showed some numbers. Later we realized that's a pulse oximeter which showed the

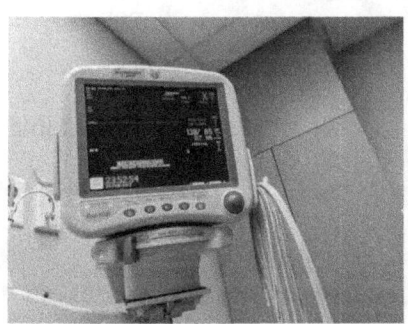 heart rate, which was very high more than 120 and SPO2 (oxygen content in the blood) which was low at around 69. The SPO2 being low was why she was unable to breathe properly. The nurse connected her to a Patient Monitor, which was

showing her SPO2 and Heart rate continuously. In the meantime, another nurse also checked her Blood Sugar, which was around 210 and was higher than normal. The first line of treatment given was to stabilize her breathing, so the nurse quickly gave her Nebulization and started her on Oxygen. Till then, the Physician In-Charge of the Casualty department came and checked my Mom and mentioned she will need to be hospitalized and said she needs to be in the ICU.

I had to replenish the items (nebulization, medications) used in the Casualty/Emergency room; pay for the time spent there and register her in the Hospital. The payment for the casualty room was on an hourly basis, so we paid for approximately one to two hours there. I went to the pharmacy to get what was to be replenished and paid for the same. Till that time, my

Mom was already moved to the ICU on the 2nd floor; I went to the Registration Desk to fill a form and make the down payment. They asked me to sign some forms which had details of next of kin/guardian names. They also asked me if I had insurance and gave me another form and told me to connect with TPA in the morning since it was already around 8.00

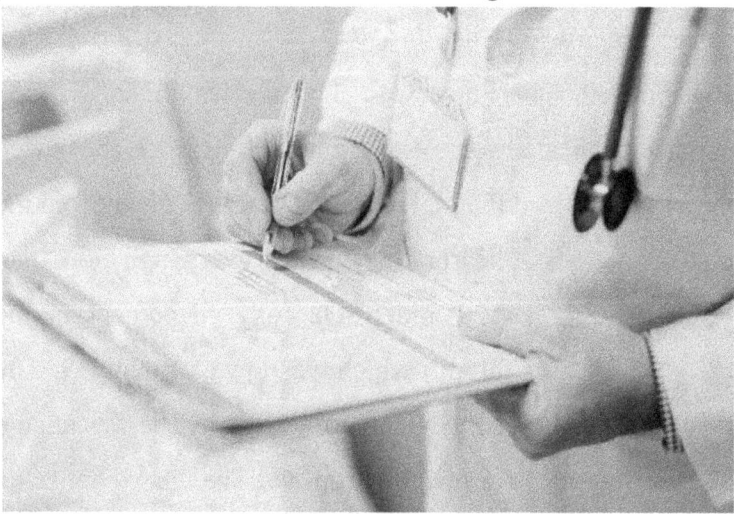

PM. The front desk employee gave me a Paper File (that also had some stickers which were Bar Codes) and two passes. She explained the use of the passes and mentioned since the patient is in the ICU, one person needs to spend the night in the hospital in the waiting area. By the time I went up, my mom had already been shifted to the ICU, so I went there with the file. The ICU was on the second floor while the casualty was on the first floor and the registration desk on the ground floor. I could go in the ICU even though it was not visiting time as I needed to talk to the Physician In-Charge. There were two Physicians present, a chest physician and a General Physician. Both were asking a lot of questions to us (me and my sister). They already ordered a CT scan and a chest X-ray which would happen probably next day and a battery of tests whose results would come in 2 hours. I mentioned we have done the X-ray and will get the film. So, I went and quickly got the film from the diagnostic center, which was 10 mins away from the Hospital.

The Physicians looked at the X-ray and mentioned: "It could be a heart or lung issue, A CT Scan will let us know what the issue is, till then, we will have to keep her on NIV." "NIV," Now, what's an NIV? The Physician mentioned it's a "Non-Invasive Ventilator." As soon as we heard Ventilator, we said No, No Ventilator. The Physician explained that it was "Non-Invasive" and that my Mom's lungs were not expanding properly; hence, she needs to use the same to get her stabilized. After this explanation, we agreed and started on the NIV machine. The nurse gave me a Paper which had a list of medications (also the Bar Code on the paper) and asked me to get the medications. I went to the hospital's Pharmacy and gave the list, the pharmacist asked me, do you have insurance? I told him, yes, but I need to give the details to the TPA department. Accordingly, he told me to pay only for the items which were not covered by the Insurance. I took the medicines to the ICU, and my mom was put on many IV (Intra-Venous) medications and Nebulizations at regular intervals. Note the Physician did not give Duolin as one of the side effects of the same is high heart rate (tachycardia).

I had to spend the night in the waiting area while my sister went to stay with my Aunt. In the ICU, there are quite a few Physicians and nurses. There's the ICU In-Charge (Main ICU Dr), 7-8 nurses depending on the number of patients. All of these come in shifts, and along with these, you also have Assigned Physicians in my mother's case, the Chest Physician and the General Physician. The Assigned Physicians come at a specific time for rounds; mostly, they come twice during a day for rounds (around 9:00 AM and 8:00 PM). The next day morning, the Physician had come for his round's things seemed fine. Most of the results had come, and everything was normal, except CO2, which was on the higher side.

One test result would come in another day, mostly, which was a Sputum Culture. The Physician mentioned we would do the CT Scan after some time. After the Scan, the Physician found that

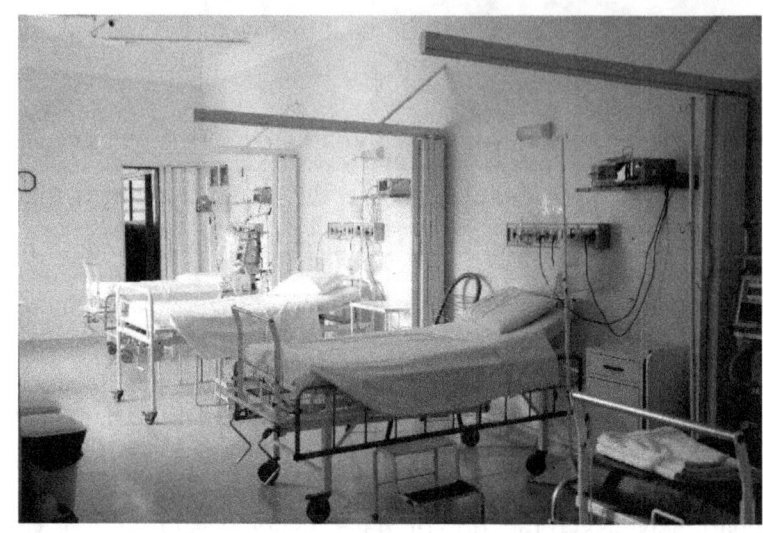

my mom had Pneumonia. The Physicians also tried to move my mom to a small Home Bi-Pap machine (like a mini ventilator), but she was not able to sustain the Oxygen (SPO2) and was moved back to the NIV. It took her couple of more days to stabilize after which she was able to sustain the SPO2 on the Home Bi-Pap machine. In between the Sputum, Culture report was also received, and we found out she had a Fungal Infection, so another medication got added to the list. Finally, after five days in the ICU, my mother was to be moved to a room and to do so, I went to the front desk for some formalities viz. choosing the type of Room. We chose a Private room, and my mom moved to the room, which was on the 6th floor. It took another couple of days after which the Physician gave a discharge. At the time of discharge, the Attending Physician prescribed my Mom to take some regular medications and continue the Home Bi-pap. She was also on O2 but based on her progress; the Physician weaned her off after some days post discharge. To monitor her progress, we had to do an ABG (Arterial blood gas) test regularly to know the CO_2 in her blood. Post my mom's discharge, we also had to keep a nurse for a few months to monitor my mother regularly and had to buy the Bi-Pap machine and keep an O2 machine handy for some time.

At the time of Discharge, I had to pay the Bill, and since I had Parental Insurance, whose details I submitted on the second day. In between the seven days, I used to go and ask how much the bill amount is. The Complete Bill was created and sent to the Insurance company via the TPA. In a couple of hours, the Insurance company asked for more details regarding the patient and why it took seven days to discharge the patient. The Hospital sent the details to the insurance company via the Hospital TPA. The Insurance company covered 70% of the entire Bill and the rest I had to Pay.

Above, was a very brief story of what happened in approximately seven days in the hospital and little before Admission and Post Discharge. So now let us try and understand the Billing cycle in this entire scenario. If we leave out the Homecare piece, the overall Cycle consists of three phases

1. What happened at the Front Desk: Front Office
2. Point of Care & Discharge: Middle Office
3. Billing: Back Office

The Patient workflow would vary in each type of case but let's try and depict the above flow in a generic manner and let's do that step by step.

Step 1 Scheduling: In a non-emergency case, one would call and schedule an appointment. Primary points which are asked by the Front Desk Employee is who is the Physician and probably the reason for the visit.

Step 2 Appointment: According to your need, the front desk employee will block the Physician's calendar and give you an Appointment.

Step 3 Pre-Registration: In case a person is coming to the hospital for a planned event like a knee replacement surgery this step will happen where the front desk employee will take more information viz Name, DOB, Insurance Details and other information.

Step 4 Insurance Eligibility: In the overall picture, this Is the first interaction between the hospital and the Insurance company. Here the hospital checks basic insurance information viz. validity of the insurance, coverage of wheelchair or ambulance. All this can be done electronically using EDI (Electronic Data Interchange), and we use EDI 270/271. We will know more about EDI in the sections ahead.

Step 5 Patient Registration: This Step and the previous step can go hand in hand; this step has a lot of Data Entry required unless the hospital is very sophisticated and uses a Tab. Primarily data entered is around Name, Address, Contact Details, Next of Kin Details, Insurance information, Medication, Family History, and quite a lot of other details.

Step 6 Patient Admission: If the Patient must stay in the Hospital, one needs to get admitted, and hence, we have another process for the same.

Step 7 Financial Counseling: This is a step which is helpful to patients by providing information regarding the Health Services, Insurance details, or Alternative Payment Methods.

All the above 7 Steps happen at the Front Desk of a Hospital; hence, they contribute towards **"The Front Office**." After this (Patient Admission) is when the main process of Care Starts, lets detail the same and put it in a structure.

Step 8 Nursing: This is a very important step in the Hospital, and it is this step which holds the Patient together throughout their journey. The nurse will attend the Patient most of the times than a physician. If you notice the nurse will come to check the vitals and other parameters before the Physician does. Even in the ICU, the nurse needs to record Patient parameters on an hourly basis. All of these constitute to form Nurse Notes.

Step 9 Physician: Post the nurse, the Physician will come and look at the Vitals and other Parameters captured. The Physician will also ask additional questions and accordingly can prescribe medications, order Lab/Path or Radiology Tests. The documentation written by the Physician constitutes to form Physician Notes.

Step 10 Medications: This is the Department which fulfills Medications ordered for Patients. This department will provide the Medication Details and how to take the same – e.g., Orally.

Step 11 Lab Order: Physicians order Laboratory Tests or Pathology exams; most big hospitals would have an in-house, Lab, or a third party is present in the premise. The Document provided by the Lab would be the Lab Results.

Step 12 Radiology Order: Similar to Lab, this Ancillary department does specific tests like X-Ray, CT Scan, MRI. The Radiology department provides Results and Inference.

Step 13 Clinical Documentation: Each of the above Steps from 8 to 12 will generate some or the other document/result/order. All of this contributes to Clinical Documentation.

Step 8 – 13 The Loop: If the Patient is there in the hospital for more than one day viz. An Inpatient the above process would be repeated number of times.

Step 14 Patient Discharge: Once the Physician feels the Patient is Fit, he/she will get a discharge. Please note this Step differs when one compares US Healthcare & Indian Healthcare. In the case of US Healthcare, the Patient receives a bill after discharge and after the Insurance has decided how much Insurance is Covered. In the case of Indian healthcare, one needs to finalize all payments on the day of the discharge.

Step 15 Medical Transcription: This is something we did not discuss earlier, but it is simply converting Written Clinical Documentation or Recorded Transcripts into Electronic Format.

Step 16 Medical Coding: This is a Step we will understand in little bit more detail, but as of now it is converting the Clinical Notes into Billing Codes where each code possibly has some Money/Billing Amount associated with it.

All the above Steps from 8 to 16 happen at the point of providing Care in the Hospital; hence, they contribute towards "**The Middle Office**." Finally, we have the Last Stage, where we calculate the billing amount.

Step 17 Charge Posting/Entry: Once the Patient is discharged, the Hospital takes 2-3 days to enter all the charges in the system. The concept of waiting for somedays is known as "Hold Days" technically; this is what can add to the AR – Accounts Receivable of the Hospital. i.e., If the Hold Days are more, the Hospital will receive Payment with more delays.

Step 18 Patient Accounting: The Patient Accounting system checks for errors within the Data, for example, someone has entered duplicate charges, or some data required for the Claim is missing. In technical terms, these errors are "Billing Edits."

Step 19 Claim File: The System will calculate the Total Bill and create the Claim File which is sent to the Payer/Insurance company directly or via a TPA (Third Party Administrator) or Clearing House. The data is sent using an EDI Transaction, and the number to keep in mind is EDI 835 called Remittance Advice.

Step 20 Claim Follow Up: If the Payer does not respond, the hospital can follow up with the Payer, and that can be again done using EDI, which is EDI 276/277.

Step 21 Payer Response: The Insurance Company will respond to the Claim File in terms of another EDI File called EDI 837 known as an Explanation of Benefits. You can compare this to any normal insurance, for example, if you have ever claimed for Car insurance, the agent tells you the Paint is not covered, this plastic & rubber is not covered, etc. Similarly, the Health Insurance company tells you XYZ medication is not covered, the procedure is not covered or partially covered.

Step 22 Hospital AR Department: The Response from the Payer can be one of the three

- A. The Claim is processed.
- B. The Claim is On Hold.
- C. Claim Denial.

In case of a denial, the Hospital can Appeal for the same; if the Claim is on hold, the Payer can ask for more information/supporting documents.

Step 23 Payment: If the Claim is processed, the hospital will receive the Payment via another EDI which EDI 820 via the Bank is.

All the above steps from 17 to 23 constitute towards "The Back Office" in Revenue Cycle Management.

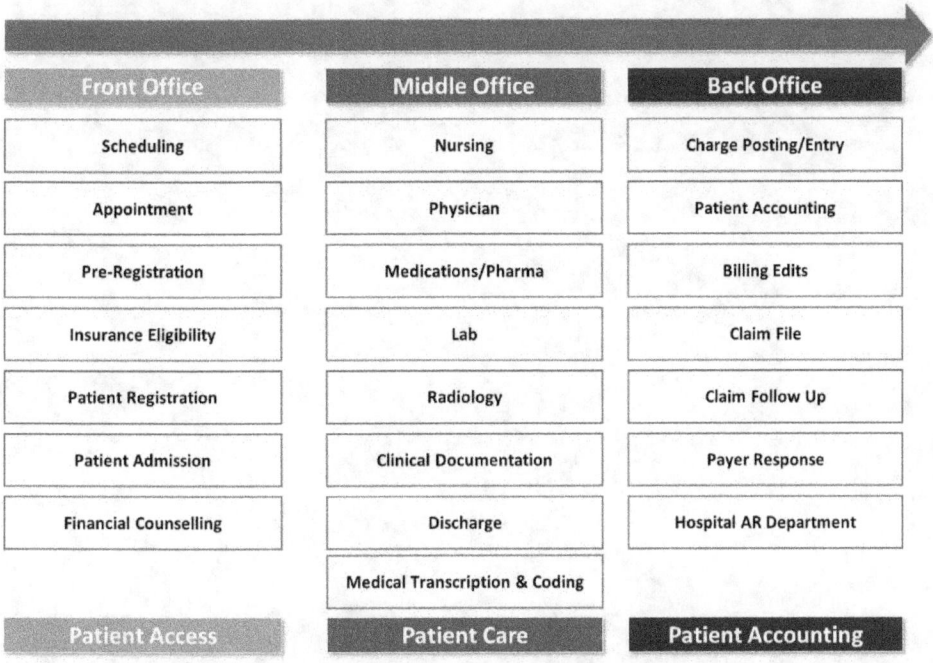

Hopefully, you are now able to relate to the three phases I mentioned earlier

1. All that happened at the Front Desk: Front Office
2. Point of Care & Discharge: Middle Office
3. Billing and Claim Processing: Back Office

#5 The Beginning of Electronic Medical Records

The concept of Electronic Medical Records / Hospital Information Systems is on the rise, but it is very intriguing to understand when Physicians start to maintain patient records. Physicians did maintain medical records, but they were more for research and publishing papers. If you have seen old movies, the Physician used to visit the patient at his/her home and give medications the Physician carries in his bag. I did not see the Physician write down anything or maintain any record per se. Documenting Medical Records came into the foray from the 1920s. Well, these were paper records. A time when patients were being treated more in hospitals than at home of the patient. The biggest challenge at that time was managing the paper records. Tabulating machines were being leveraged by

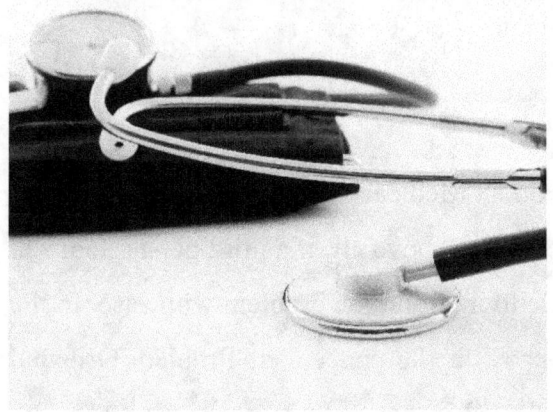

hospitals to manage paper records. One of the earliest machines used was the "Hollerith Tabulating Machine."

Till this point, there wasn't any standard methodology to document Patient Medical Records. Let us try and understand the details of how can we document this data (Medical Records). Let us say a Patient ABC comes to the hospital complaining of a stomachache; the patient fills the forms waits for the nurse to come. The nurse comes and asks basic questions and documents the details asked on a Paper; these constitute as Nurse Notes. After which the Physician comes asks some more questions and documents the details – these constitute as Physician notes.

The Physician prescribes medications, Lab Test, and an X-Ray. The Patient goes to the Lab to do the test's – at the end, the patient gets the Lab 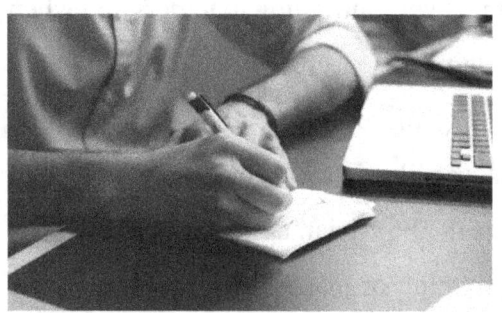 Results. Similarly, the Radiologist would provide the X-Ray and results. All these data elements, together, will form the Medical Record, but there is a twist. From a Physician's point of view, these are Source Oriented Medical Records. Any guesses why? Cause they are organized from the source where it was created

1.   Nurse Notes
2.   Physician Notes/Progress Notes
3.   All Lab Results
4.   All X-Ray Results

The data is good in terms of a Patient Medical Record, but it does not help track a problem which the patient has. Above all, if a third person looks at the data, he/she might not be able to interpret the problem with ease. In the 1960s, Dr. Larry Weed came up with the concept of Problem-Oriented Medical Records (POMR). Dr. Weed in his lectures mentions that some Physicians ask five questions and some fifty-five; he emphasized that the questions should be around on Branching Logic and in 9 minutes one can gather a lot of Patient information. Overall, he mentioned that there are 4 phases of a POMR

1. Maintain a Database – This has the Patients history, Physical and Lab Work, etc.
2. A Problem List
3. Plan for each problem
4. Follow up Plan – Titled and Numbered Progress Notes.

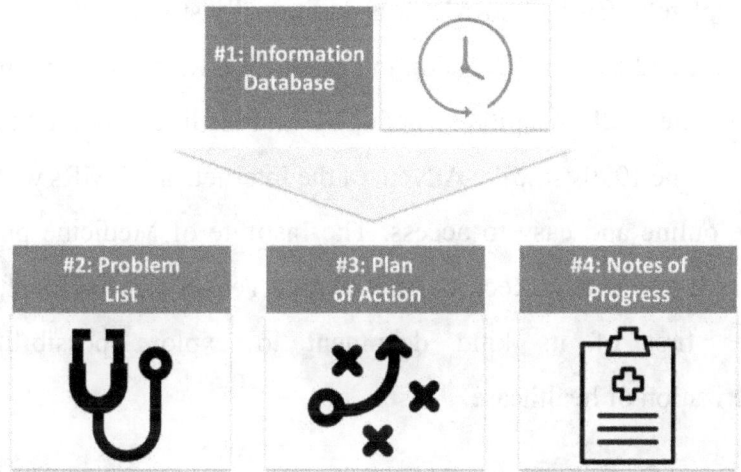

Medical Records came into the picture to help in maintaining Patient History, but another reason for their rise is they help in Audits, medical litigation (which saw an increase in the 1960s) and for health insurance to decide rates and denials. As per the practical experience of Physicians, POMR was time-consuming. After POMR, came the concept of SOAP notes, which was an improved version of the same. In this case, "S" stands for Subjective which has details of the Patients Current Condition (Medical & Surgical History, Family & Social History). "O" stands for Observation/Objective which contains details of the Patient Vitals, Lab Tests and other observations. "A" stands for Assessment which is the Medical Diagnosis for that visit, and "P" for Plan, which is the Treatment

Plan. This clinical documentation (in whatever format POMR or SOAP) helps the Medical Coders in entering the appropriate ICD code for billing purposes.

In the 1970s, Regenstrief Medical Record (RMR) one of the initial EMRs was developed by McDonald & associates and Indiana University School of Medicine. Wishard Memorial Hospital in Indianapolis was using RMR. The RMR was complementary to the paper records not replacing the same completely. By 1977, RMR was additionally storing Lab Results, X-Ray studies, and ECG's. The adoption rate of EMRs during this time was very low, but still, hospital scheduling and billing were done using computers. The 1990s saw the Advent of the Internet, and EMRs were made available online and easy to access. The Institute of Medicine published Computer-Based Patient Record: An Essential Technology for Health Care, this was first of its kind document to explore possibilities of computerization of healthcare.

The document focused on different attributes (12 in total) such as Problem List, Clinical Reasoning, Data Entry, Clinical Problem Solving. The recommendation was for all Physicians to use Computers to Improve Patient Care. 1996 saw a New law coming into the picture in to deal with growing issues of Security and Privacy known as HIPAA. Feb 2009 brought a new law to not only implementing an EMR but also to Meaningfully use the EMR. Hospitals are currently in 2018-19 trying to implement EMRs and meaningfully use them :-)

As of now, there are so many EMR/EHR systems, some of the top Market Leaders are EPIC, Meditech, Cerner which are for Inpatients. The Inpatient EMR systems each have separate modules for Admission, Billing,

Insurance Eligibility, and each step for that matter. Then there are specific ones for Specialties viz Sunquest Lab, GE Radiology and even for Bed Tracking provided by Teletracking. It is not necessary that a Hospital would have only one type of EMR/EHR they could be using different modules at different steps. For example, a hospital can have Meditech ADT, which is for admissions, EPIC Resolute HB for hospital Billing, and EPIC PB for Physician Billing. I have tried to depict the below image showcasing different modules of Meditech.

Most of the Meditech modules have a three-character acronym, for example in the Clinical and Ancillary systems we have BBK which is known as Blood bank, LAB for Laboratory and POM for order entry.

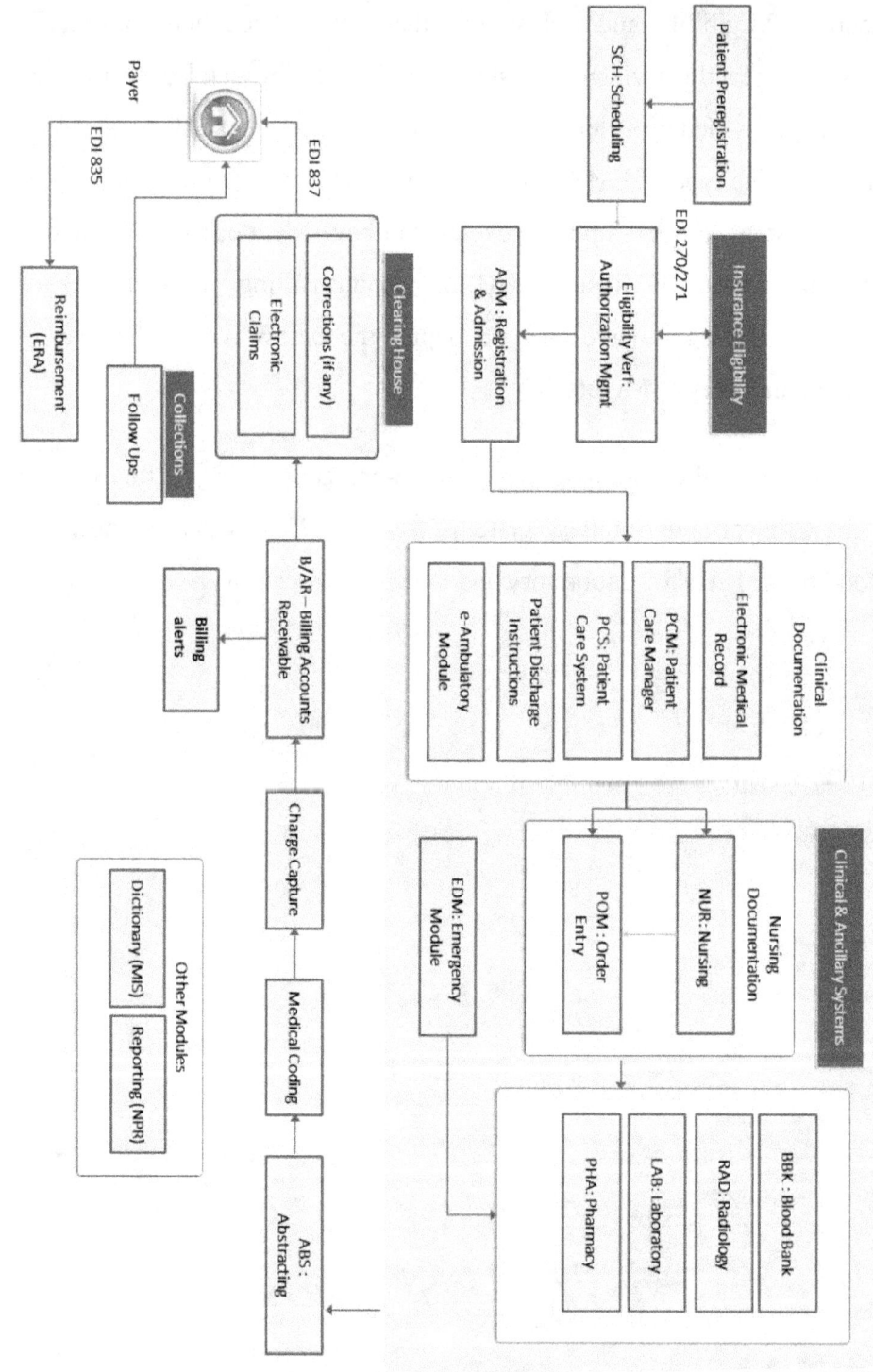

#6 The Tidal Wave of Regulations

Regulation is a Law or an official rule to control a specific activity. Overall Healthcare has seen a lot of regulations come in over the years. In the earlier sections, we talked about how the UB-04 form came into existence. In the prior section, we briefly also talked about HIPAA and Meaningful use of EHR. There are many regulations, but I am talking more about some of the regulations which impact the IT systems. If you know a little history, the Internet first came into existence in 1969. In 1969 an experiment was done to connect two entities "Stanford University" and the "University of California." TCP/IP was the protocol for ARPANET in 1982. TCP/IP was the basis of the Internet becoming a reality, and the world slowly started to connect.

Jon Romney & Simon Hackett first connected a Sunbeam Deluxe Toaster to the Internet in 1990 at the Interop conference. At this time, there were only 310K computers in the world, and only 1.3million people had access to the internet. If you notice the IT trend, one of the first systems which were automated or made electronic were supply chain and finance. In the healthcare industry, Finance/Billing areas were the first to use IT. EMR systems have been in the market since the 1970s but have picked up pace in recent times. Even HIMSS (Health Information and Management Systems Society) has defined their own 8 (0 to 7) phases of how a hospital can become completely Electronic. Let us quickly look at the Phases/Steps.

Stage 0: Stage 0 implies no Ancillaries implemented in the hospital, which includes the Lab Information System, Radiology Information System, and Pharmacy System

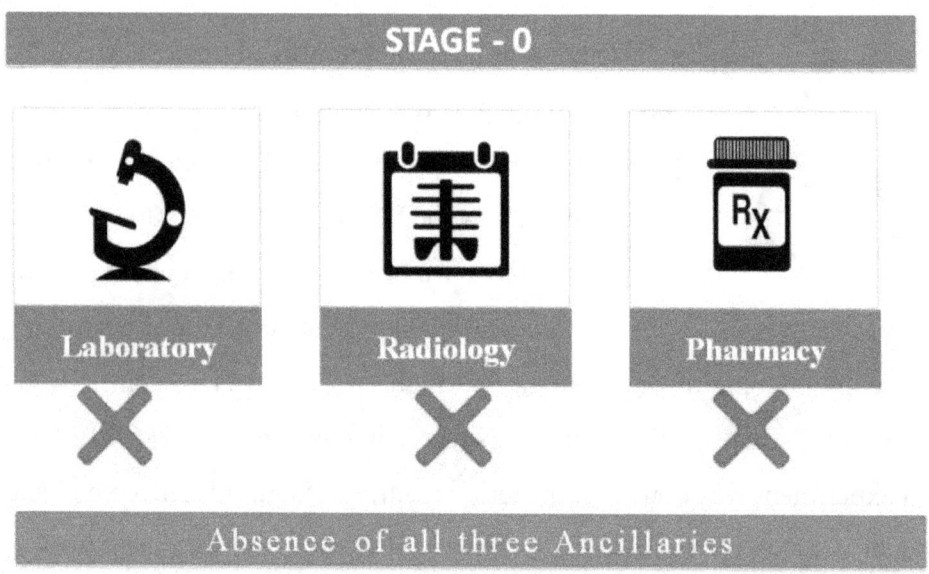

Stage 1: Software's for all three Ancillaries are installed in the hospital, but they don't talk to each other.

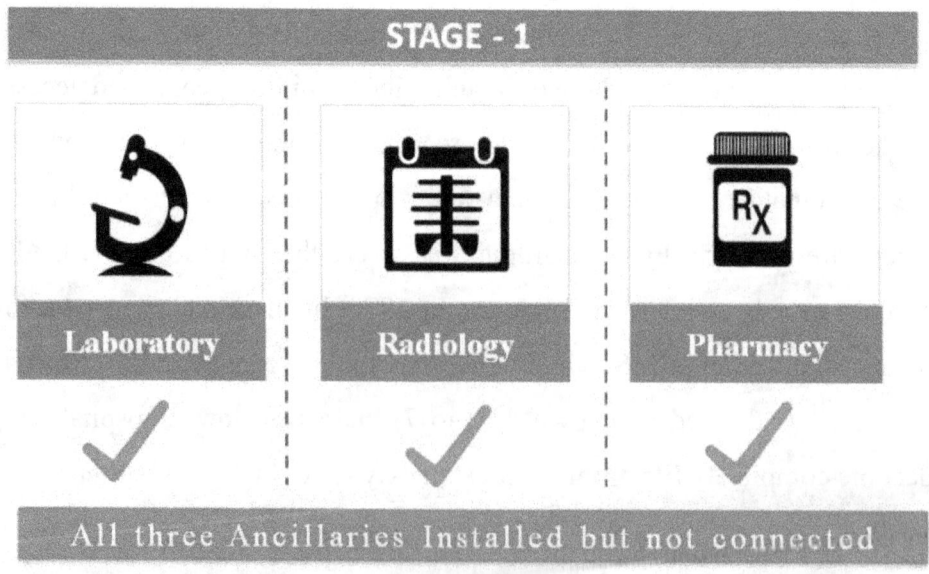

Stage 2: All three Ancillaries have been implemented and are interconnected

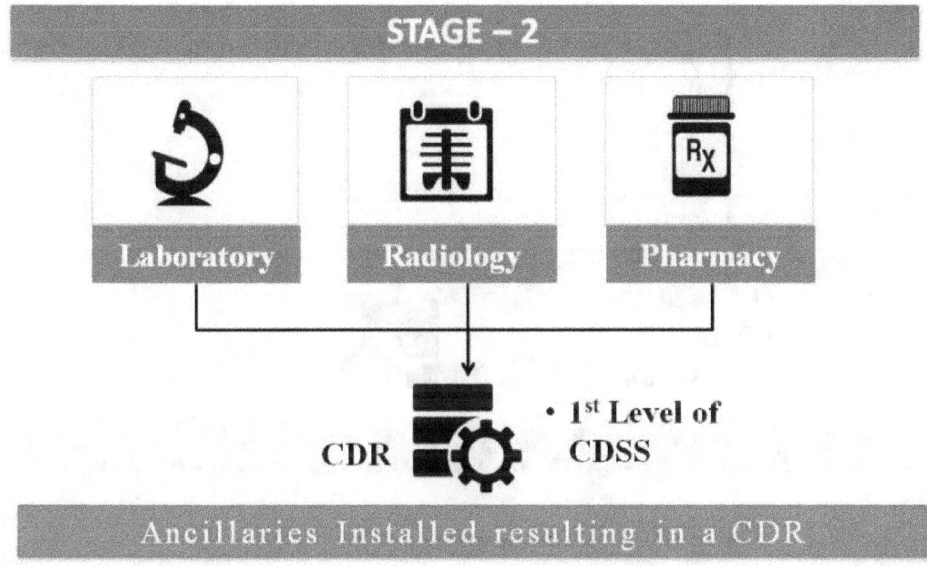

Stage 3: Other Systems are implemented viz Clinical Documentation, eMAR, nursing

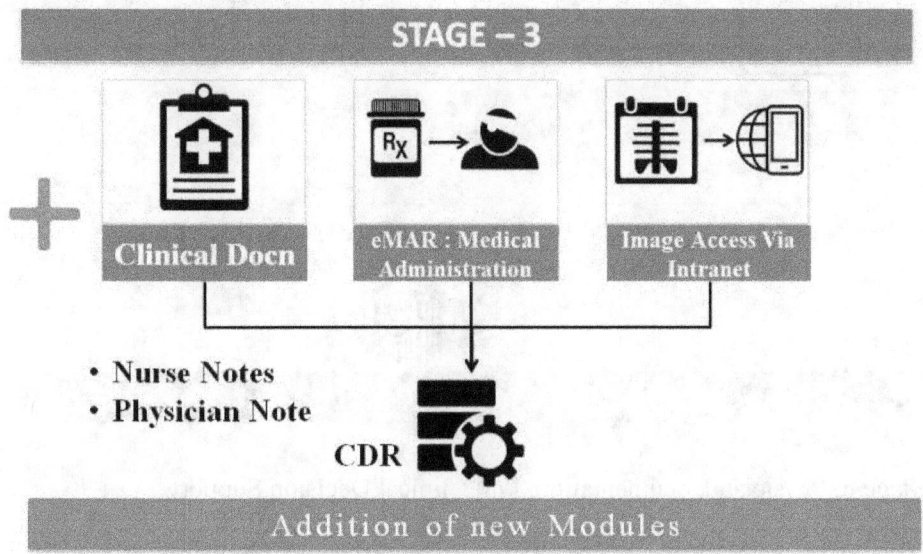

Stage 4: Addition of CPOE & Clinical Decision Support

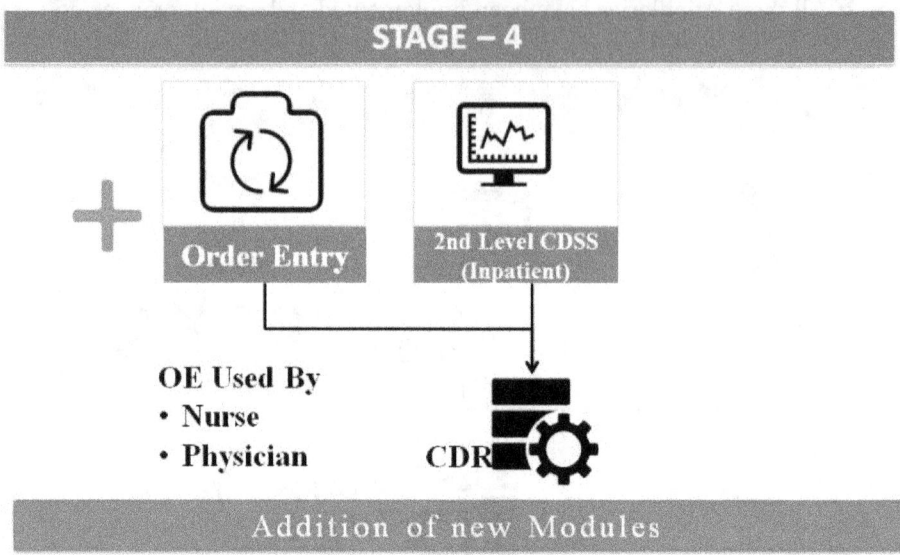

Stage 5: Closed Loop Medical Administration

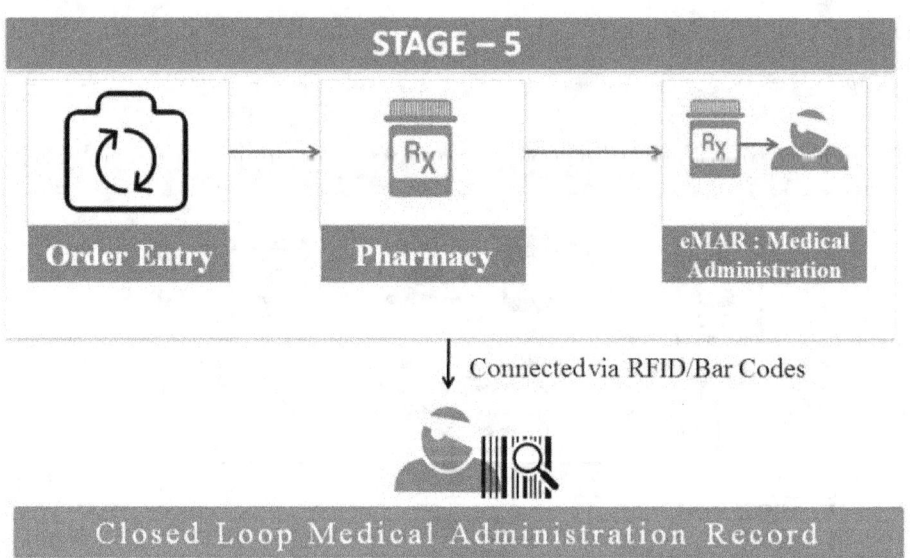

Stage 6: Physician Documentation, Full Clinical Decision Support

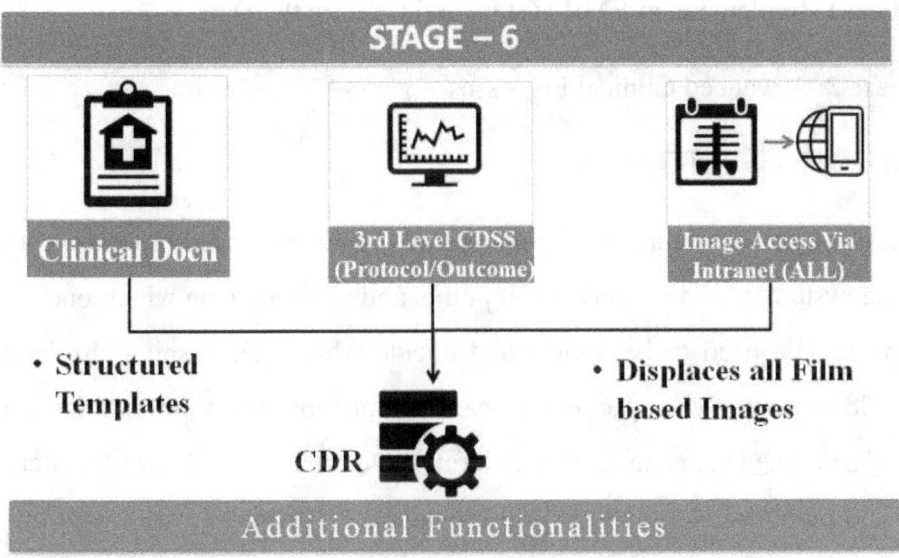

Stage 7: Complete EMR; CCD transactions to share data

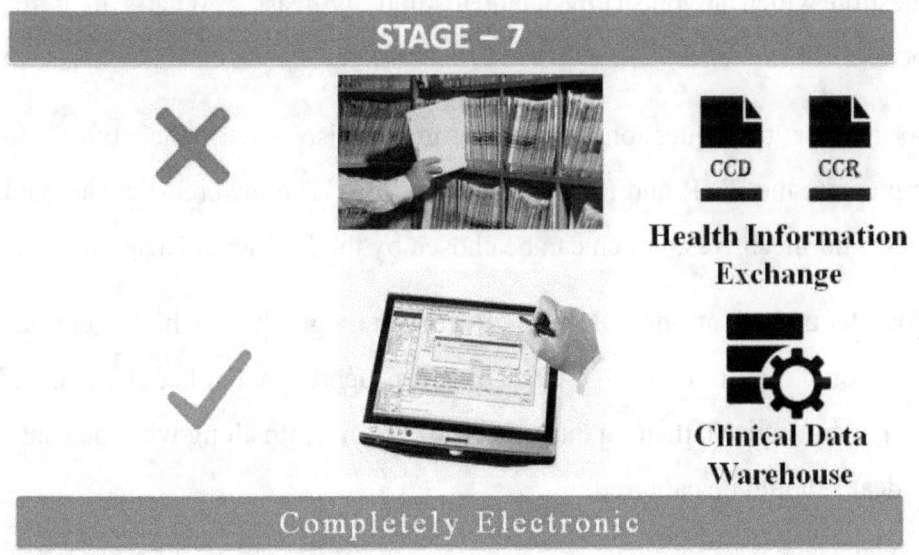

As mentioned earlier in Feb 2009, a new law was bought in to not only implementing an EMR but also to Meaningfully use the EMR. It is like an Exam which you need to give if you are capturing the data and also using it well or not. Meaningful use consists of three stages

Phase 1: Implement an EMR system and Capture the Data

Phase 2: Advanced Clinical Processes

Phase 3: Improved Outcomes

But what kind of data would you capture, as we discussed in the revenue cycle system, we saw many touch points and so much data which one can capture. We need to be logical and decide what each hospital/physician should capture in each phase. One can look at capturing simple things like Vitals, Active Diagnosis Codes, Allergies, Demographics. Now the criteria should be different for Eligible Physicians and Hospitals, along with this, there also should be some mandatory criterion (CORE), and for some which one can make a choice (MENU). All these criteria are fine, but the main question which anyone (Physician/Hospital) will ask, "What's in it for me/us?"

To answer this question, the government also gave "Incentives" to implement the EMR and to use it meaningfully. There were Medicare and Medicaid Incentives, which can be chosen by the Physician/Hospital.

Now, let us look at one criterion – Record demographics, which mentions one should capture Language, Date of Birth, Gender, and other elements. If the patient expired, then, in that case, the date of death along with the cause of death should be captured.

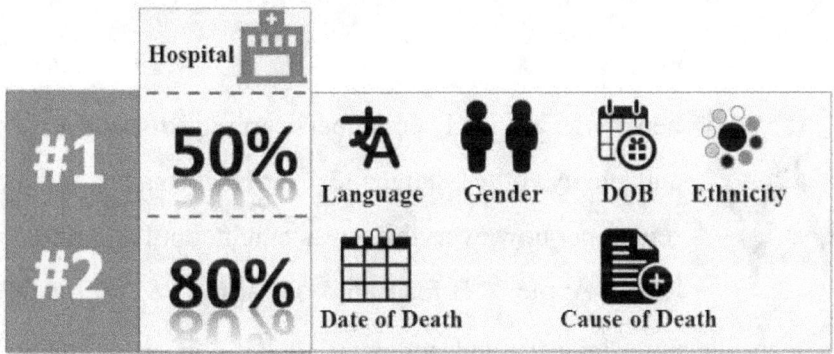

The image gives the details; you will see some number, #1 means Stage 1, while #2 indicates Stage 2. So, what the measure mentions is that in Stage 1 for 50% of the patients that come into the hospital, one should capture their demographics, while in Stage 2, the number goes to 80%.

Similar lines, there are many other Regulations around Accountable Care Organization, Implementation of ICD-10, and there definitely could be one in the future around ICD-11.

#7 How to Speak Healthcare

When I was a Kid, I remember learning to speak English and many other languages for that matter. I don't remember how everything was taught, but I do remember "A for Apple," "B for Ball," "C for Cat" & "D for Dog" ☺. On a similar note, let's try and understand what I mean by "How to Speak Healthcare." The word Speak is more in the context of how a computer can understand Healthcare Terminology, known as terminology standards.

Let me give an example; the Physician says Patient X has got Asthma; in general, most people would understand what the Physician is saying. But the Computer understands numbers 1's and 0's. Hence for the Computer to understand, we need numbers. To understand healthcare data, we have Concepts like Diagnosis Codes called ICD – International Classification of diseases now being owned by the WHO (World Health Organization). ICD-10 is a number; for example, J45.901 represents Asthma, which would be easy for the computer to understand. Oh, by the way, ICD-10 is the 10th version of ICD.

One of the early references of systematically classifying diseases goes back to 1800s by William Farr (in 1837) a British Statistician and Jacques Bertillon (in 1893) who was a French Statistician. Before that, François Bossier de Lacroix, a French Physician, tried to do the same in the 1700s. All of them were trying to Analyze statistics related to death and disease. Bertillon introduced the "Bertillon Classification of Causes of Death" in

1893. It was in 1946 when the United Nations asked WHO to take over the responsibility of revision of the statistics which became ICD. The 9th version was out in the late 1970s, and the 10th version came out in 1990.

ICD-10 has two components one for Diagnosis (ICD-10-CM Diagnosis Codes, ~68,000 codes) and another for procedures (ICD-10 Procedure Coding System, ~87,000 codes).

Similar lines, we also have SNOMED-CT, which is called "Systematized Nomenclature of Medicine – Clinical Terms," and it is a huge collection of Medical terms—over 300,000 active concepts. SNOMED is clinically very rich and is fast becoming the preferred terminology for Analytics to provide better decision support, quality measures (PQRI), and disease management. Above all, SNOMED also has concepts related to Symptoms and findings. Along with this, SNOMED also has an underlying map to convert SNOMED to ICD-10.

The above codes we spoke about were for Diagnosis and Procedure Codes viz ICD-9, ICD-10, or SNOMED-CT. But the hospital environment is just not limited to Diagnosis; you have medicines, medical equipment, Lab Results, and so many other elements.

Most commonly used Codes for Medicines are NDC – National Drug Code, NDF-RT - National Drug File - Reference Terminology. US FDA created NDC, and the Federal Register of 2nd July 1969 mentions the following

"The National Drug Code System will provide an identification system in computer language to permit automated processing of drug data by Government agencies, drug manufacturers and distributors, hospitals, and insurance companies."

As per the Federal Register agreement and National Drug Code (NDC) would consist of a nine-character code. As of now, the codes are 10 to 11 digits.

- The first three characters are the Labeler Identity Code assigned by the Food and Drug Administration. As of now, these are four characters.
- The next four characters are the Drug Product Identity Code
- The last two characters are the Trade Package Identity Code, are assigned by the drug firms within parameters defined by the FDA.

The below image gives the NDC code for Prozac created by Dista Products, and it comes in a package of 100 capsules.

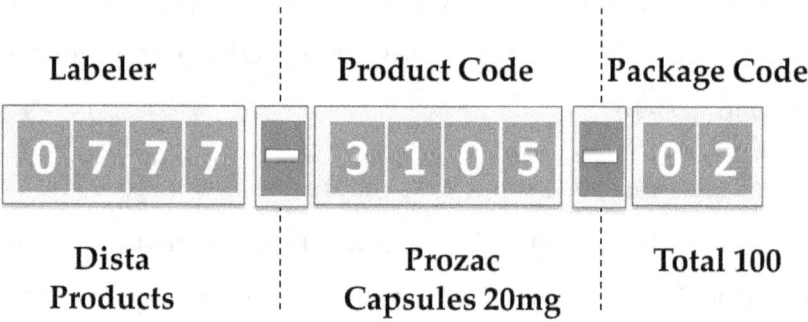

Similarly, the NDC code 0555-0483-02 indicates "Amiloride Hydrochloride and Hydrochlorothiazide" (0483) manufactured by Teva Pharmaceuticals (0555) and comes as 100 tablets in a bottle.

We also have another set of codes to identify medications which are called as RXNorm and was developed in 2001 by NLM – National Library for Medicine. The key purpose for the same was to improve the interoperability of drug terminology.

RxCUI	RxNorm Name
208558	Ticlid 250 MG Oral Tablet
313406	Ticlopidine 250 MG Oral Tablet

Then you have medical equipment's which also need to be coded, for which we use HCPCS (Healthcare Common Procedure Coding System) also pronounced as "Hick-Picks." CMS developed HCPCS for reporting medical procedures and services. Using HCPCS was made mandatory from 1996 as per HIPAA.

- Level I codes consist of the CPT (Common Procedural Terminology) codes and are numeric. Example
- Level II codes are the HCPCS alphanumeric code set and primarily include non-physician products, supplies, and procedures not included in CPT. E.g., Ambulance services and prosthetic devices.

Finally, we have LOINC Codes which identify health measurements, observations, and documents.

LOINC_NUM	LOINC Fully Specified Name
49689-3	Glucose tolerance [Interpretation] in Serum or Plasma Narrative--post 100 g glucose PO
2345-7	Glucose [Mass/volume] in Serum or Plasma
2160-0	Creatinine [Mass/volume] in Serum or Plasma

By the way, LOINC is Logical Observation Identifiers Names and Codes and was developed in 1994 by Clem McDonald who was working at Regenstrief Institute then.

#8 How to Write Healthcare

Now that we know how to speak some Healthcare, let's see how we could write a little Healthcare. Let's take a simple example many times a Physician will prescribe a Lab or Radiology Test on a prescription pad. The patient will take the paper prescription to the Lab Technician and get the test done and wait for the result. The patient will take the results and take it to the Physician for discussion/analysis. Now when I say Write, I want to reduce most of the manual intervention (take the prescription or the results) that would happen and do everything electronically. That is where we use Standards, and in this case, Technology standards and writing is "Data Transmission." The simplest example which I could give in today's world is an Email, which is a Data Transmission Standard.

Let's look an analogy here which you can probably relate. I Assume most of you have been to McDonald's and order a burger. The person taking the order is not writing down something on a chit and giving it to the cook. He is just putting the data in his computer, and it flashes on the screen where the food is cooking. Based on the pipeline, you get your order once ready. Let us look at the example of Dr. Janish giving a Prescription for some Lab tests to Mr. Alphonso Robert. Mr. Alphonso has been asked to do a CBC (complete blood count), Creatinine, and Blood Sugar Fasting.

If you are not aware of these tests, let me give a small explanation. CBC is normally one of the first diagnostic tests done to check various problems like anemia, infection, etc. Creatinine is done to check how well your kidneys are functioning, and Blood Sugar Fasting is done to check how well your body is managing blood sugar.

In this case, we don't want Mr.

ZNVille Hospital
ZNV Area, CV, Zip Code 27393

Mr. Alphonso Robert   29th June 2017
36 years

CBC
Blood Sugar
Creatine

Dr. Janish M
M.B.B.S, MS (SURG.) FAIS, FMAS

ZNV Area, CV, Zip Code 27393
phone: +555-456-7890
Email: info@email.com

Alphonso to take a paper prescription to the Diagnostic center; we want to send this electronically. We can send an email with details, but it would be free text and not structured, which is why we have standards like HL7, CCD, and others. But how do I convert this prescription into an HL7 standard?

1. HL7 (Health Level Seven):

First, let us look at what is HL7, HL7 stands for Health level seven it has been there for quite some time now (Late 1980s early 1990s) and has various versions. Versions can be compared to be something similar to Windows versions; each version has a new feature. HL7 is designed to capture all possible real-world events which would happen within the hospital. For example, if a patient comes to the hospital for registration, admission, discharge, or transfer his data has needs to be captured accordingly and sent to other departments. HL7 can support all these interactions between different departments with ease.

Now, let's come back to Mr. Alphonso; let us try and group some of the data elements on the prescription.

The prescription has data which is used to identify Mr. Alphonso who is the patient, in this case, here we have

- Patient Information
  - First Name
  - Last Name
  - Age

We also have information about the Hospital and the Physician which includes the following

- Hospital Information
  - Hospital Name
  - Address, State & Zip Code
- Physician Information
  - First Name
  - Last Name

Finally, we have the diagnostic tests which the Physician has ordered for the patient.

- Lab Orders
  - CBC
  - Blood Sugar Fasting
  - Creatinine

We want to send all this data directly to the Diagnostic center rather than Mr. Alphonso taking the paper prescription. In HL7 technical parlance, a Lab Test order is a Trigger Event; in other words, a real-world event. You can compare it to ordering something online nowadays, using a food delivery App. Once you order something, you get an acknowledgment in response. HL7 also works in the same way; Lab Test is the Trigger event based on which one would send the order details to the diagnostic lab, and in return, one would get acknowledgment.

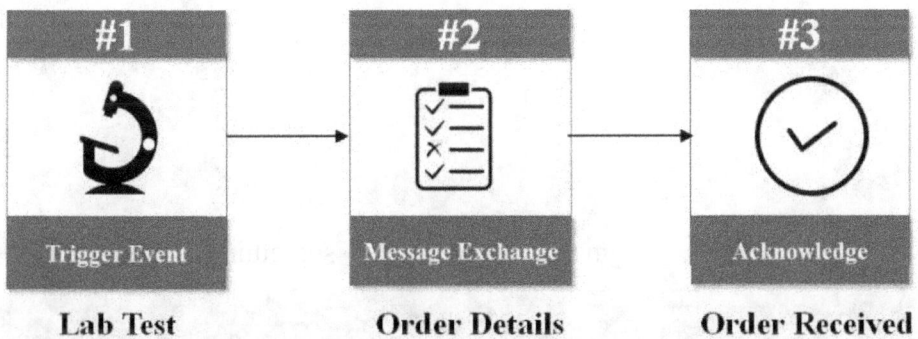

Now we have all the information grouped by logical areas, and that is how we send them. Each logical area is called a segment, again in HL7 parlance Patient Information is called as Patient Identification and represented as three characters PID. Similarly, Physician Information will fall under Patient Visit represented by PV1 and Diagnostic orders fall under Observation Request represented by OBR segment.

The below image shows how the PID segment will look like for the Lab Order when put together, you will see a lot of pipes (blue background boxes) and carrots (green background box), but you need not bother about those. Just try and see if you can see the relevant information in the jungle of pipes.

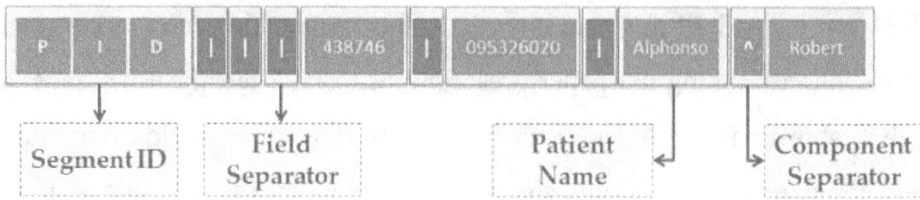

The PV1 segment would look something like below

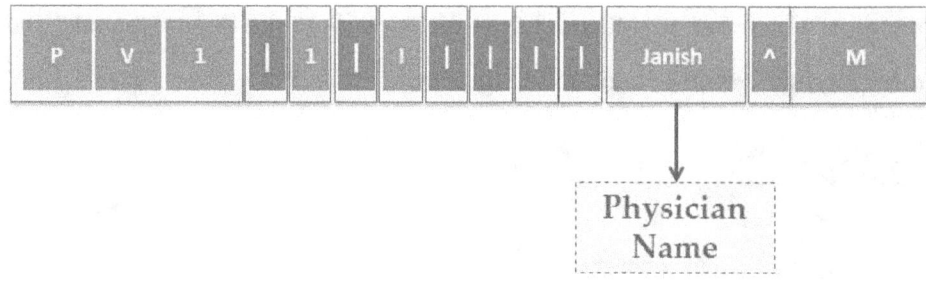

While the OBR segment will look something like below.

Please, note each orange box has a meaning, but I am not getting into those details as it is highly technical, and I don't want to bore you guys ☺. Overall when you put all segments together, the message will look something like below. Hopefully, I have not scared you all, it looks complicated, but it isn't that complicated ☺

```
MSH|^~\&|HIS|ZnVille|LIS|ZnVille
|20180101||ORM^O01|MSGID10|P|2.3
PID|||12001||Alphonso^Robert^^^Mr.||19820824|M|||West
St.^^Denver^CO^80020^USA|||||||
PV1||1|||||Janish^M|||OP
ORC|NW|20190307110114
OBR|1|20190307110114||85027^CBC (Complete Blood Count)
OBR|2|20190307110114||82565^Creatinine
OBR|3|20190307110114||82947^Fasting Blood Sugar
```

Overall, we spoke about all the information and how we can send the same using HL7. But we also need to send one more information in the message. I know I am sending information regarding Lab Orders, but the computer also needs to understand what am I sending. For this we have the Message Header viz. the MSH segment, if you notice in the header, I have highlighted three specific elements. First being ORM which is telling you that this is a General Order Message, O01 is the trigger event indicating the information given will be related to a new order or updates to existing order. Finally, you see a number 2.3 which tells you the version of HL7.

So, that is how HL7 works in a very brief manner; hopefully, I have not complicated things for you ☺.

2. **EDI (Electronic Data Interchange):**

EDI is also known as paperless trading, like HL7, EDI is used for "computer to computer" transfer of routine documents between organizations. The benefit being you are using a standard way of communication.

EDI was initially created for Supply chain systems for the interaction of two different entities Viz. Purchase Orders and Invoices. I assume everyone has bought something at least once online. In today's world, you can go to Amazon search for something like a watch, book, or any other item. You like the watch; you can check out the watch and pay for the item using a Payment gateway. Once you make the payment your order is shipped to your address. Pretty simple right?

That's not how transactions were done in the 1960s & 1970s, instead of one of us buying something let us take the example of ZNVille Hospital trying to buy Syringes and other medical equipment in bulk from SYZMakers & Co. To place an order, ZNVille creates a Purchase Order Form/Document like below.

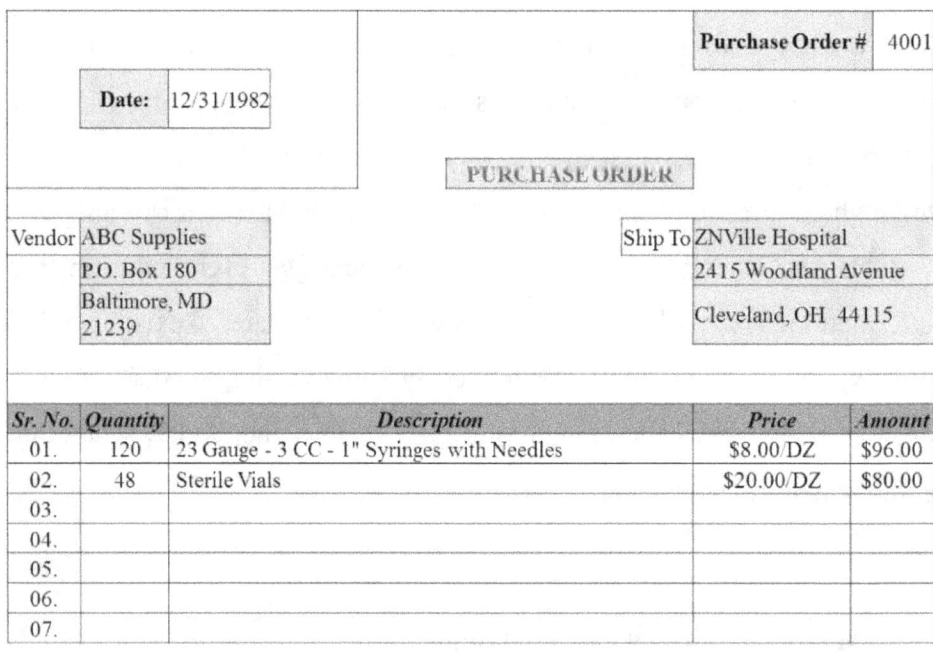

This document gives details of the Vendors Name and address, along with this, it also gives the shipping address for ZNVille hospital. You will also notice line items with order details. In this case, ZNVille has ordered for

120 "Syringes with Needles" and 48 "Sterile Vials" along with the price per dozen. This Purchase order can be handwritten or printed, and SYZMakers will receive the Purchase order by Post. Yes, you read that correctly, Via the Post Office.

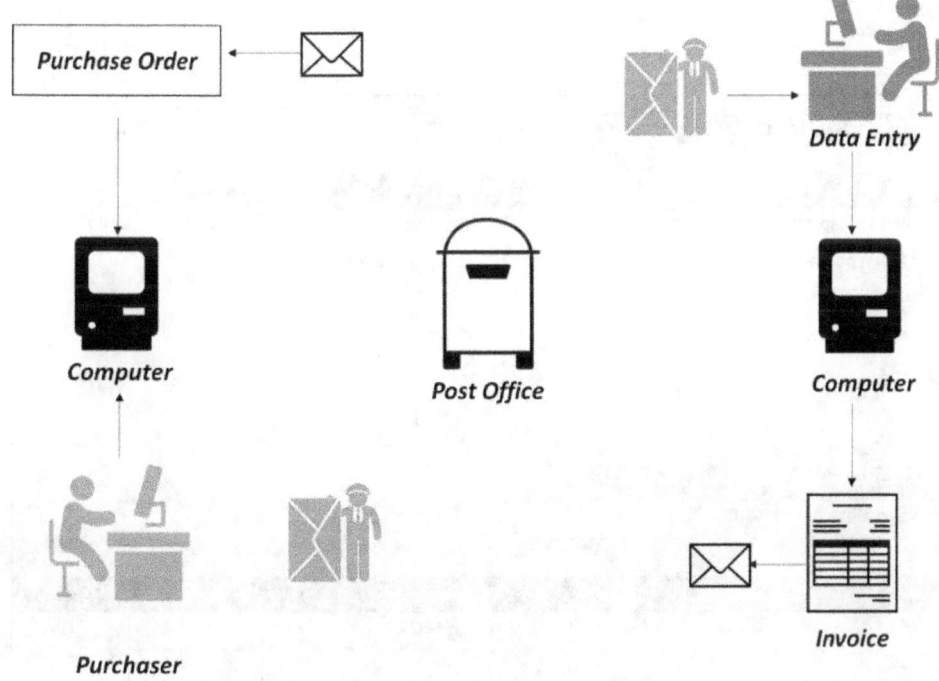

Figure: Old Way of Doing Business

The postman would deliver the purchase order to SYZMakers; in turn, SYZMakers would create an Invoice like below. ZNVille Hospital will receive the invoice along with the supplies. In simple words, EDI helps make this process completely electronic. So, in the current scenario, the process becomes very simple as one can send across a Purchase Order via an EDI 850 and receive an Invoice via and EDI 810.

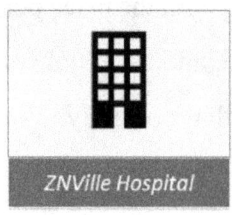 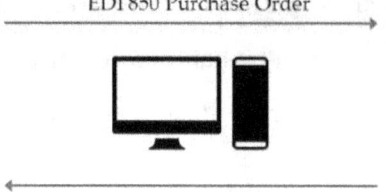 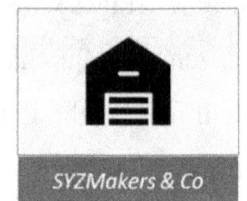

EDI 850 Purchase Order

ZNVille Hospital

SYZMakers & Co

EDI 810 Invoice

SYZMakers & Co

INVOICE

BILL TO:	**SHIP TO:**	**DATE:**	1/10/83
ZNVille Hospital	ZNVille Hospital	**INVOICE #**	14001
2415 Woodland Avenue	2415 Woodland Avenue	**Customer ID**	112
Cleveland, OH 44115	Cleveland, OH 44115		

SALESPERSON	P.O. #	SHIP DATE
Shawn Beta	4001	1/10/83

ITEM #	DESCRIPTION	QTY	UNIT PRICE	TOTAL
2343	23 Gauge - 3 CC - 1" Syringes with Needles	120	1.00	120.00
3456	Sterile Vials	48	1.67	80.00
				-
				-

SUBTOTAL	$ 200.00
TAX RATE	6.875%
TAX	$ 13.75
S & H	$ -
OTHER	$ -
TOTAL	**$ 213.75**

Other Comments or Special Instructions

1. Total payment due in 30 days
2. Kindly include the invoice number on your check

All checks payable to
SYZMakers & Co

Any questions regarding this invoice, please contact
Shawn Beta Ph [239-473-8829]

The overall process becomes simpler as it reduces a lot of paperwork, thereby reducing manual errors. One would also have a faster turnaround times and decreased mailing costs. Now, in Healthcare, there are other EDI transactions. By the way, do note in EDI the three numbers like 850 or 810 give details of the EDI transaction. The three numbers are similar to HL7, where OML refers to General Order message.

So, we understand, EDI is a standard/structure defined to send specific data in a specific format from one computer to another between two entities. Also, all entities who do business using EDI are Trading Partners. Coming back to the Healthcare transactions, just listing a few as we will see more when we talk about HIPAA.

EDI	Transaction Set
EDI 837	Health Care Claim Transaction set
EDI 835	Health Care Claim Payment/Advice Transaction Set
EDI 834	Benefit Enrollment and Maintenance Set

3. CCR/CCD:

The next format is CCD/CCR; Well if you are thinking CCD is Café Coffee Day you are very much mistaken ☺. CCD means **Continuity of Care Document** while CCR means Continuity of Care Record. A new format, CDA, is mandated by Meaningful Use, which is a combination of the best features of CCD and CCR, is proposed. It is known as C-CDA Consolidated Clinical Documentation Architecture.

The difference between HL7 and CCD is that HL7 is more transactional. HL7 can mimic almost every interaction within the hospital; there are almost more than 50 types of ADT (Admit Discharge Transfer) trigger events. In contrast, CCD is a compact format of the data; it will give you the history of the patient, and all encounters the patient would have had till date. In short, it is a snapshot in time with the core facts of the patient. As mentioned earlier, we now use CCDA within which you have the sections of CCD, there are many sections of CCD, but I am listing a few of them.

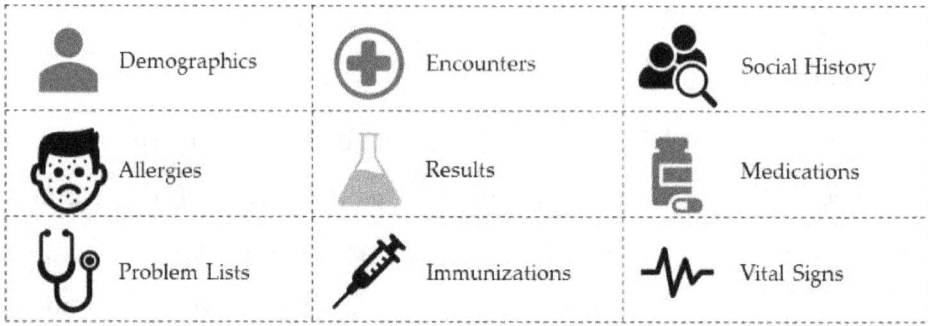

The image is self-explanatory, but a quick one-liner for each of them should help you out.

a. **Demographics**: Contains details of the patients age, gender, language, address and contact details.

b. **Encounters:** Contains details of prior encounters of the patient with the hospital. Each encounter can have information related to the visit date, Chief complaint, Height, Weight, and patient diagnosis.

c. **Social History**: Contains information related to some of the questions asked by the nurse in the like do you smoke, drink, or exercise for that matter.

d. **Allergies**: Contains details of possible allergies the patient has viz food allergy or substance allergy along with the possible start date of the allergy.

e. **Results**: Contains details of all Tests the Patient would have undergone till now viz Hemoglobin, Creatinine, Chest X-Ray along with the result and observation.

f. **Medications**: Contains details of all medications the patient would have taken in all encounters. Example, the patient, is on Betaloc 50 for hypertension

g. **Problem Lists**: Contains details of Active problems the patient has like Hypertension, Diabetes, etc.

h. **Immunizations**: Contains details of vaccines which the patient would have taken and on which day/date. E.g., Patient took the Influenza virus vaccine on 1st Jan 2019.

i. **Vital Signs**: Contains details of vitals of the patient viz. height, weight, and blood pressure.

CCDA format is in XML, and it does not look so appealing hence I am showing the output of a CCDA viewer which can make it easy for you to understand the data. The output is that of MaxMD Direct CCDA Viewer. The output shows you details of various areas, and I have just expanded allergies and immunizations.

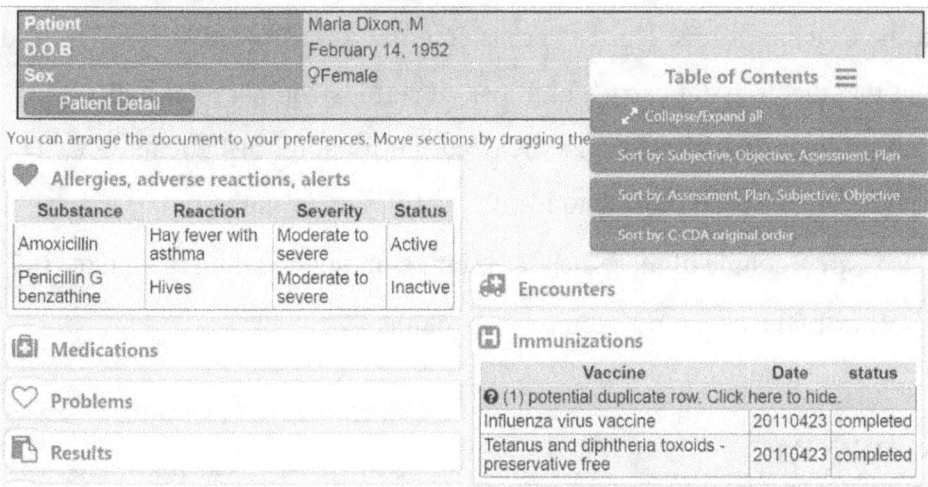

Now, let us try and understand where CCD can be leveraged. In 2012, there was a very good article published in the American Journal of Public Health around the use of CCD. The article demonstrates specific examples/areas where CCD has been used in the past and accordingly demonstrate the potential of CCD. I have mentioned a summary of a couple of examples of how CCD data can support Population Health Analysis.

Example 1: This gives information as to how we can capture data for Diabetes, which is a chronic disease impacting more than 20 million lives. As part of the initiative to monitor Diabetes, it is mandatory to report HbA1c which is **Glycosylated Hemoglobin**

Organizations can use EHR's systems to send data in CCD format. Using CCD as a transmission format can help reduce the reporting burden, and this can extend the Analytics to other chronic diseases as well like Hypertension.

Example 2: The second example talks about the use of Vioxx/rofecoxib, which was to treat chronic pain with any significant side effects. But in 2004 the drug was removed from the market due to safety concerns as it seemed to be causing deaths. Kaiser Permanente did a retrospective study to find out that the drug did carry a high risk of serious coronary heart disease. In similar lines, one can analyze the death information of Patients in CCD's and do ongoing monitoring to identify similar cases in the future.

There are a couple of more standards but, I am not detailing them like HL7, CCD or EDI as it would become too technical ☺.

4. DICOM:

Have you ever got an X-Ray done? You might get a standard Chest X-Ray done If you are doing an Annual Check-Up. In my case, I had to get an X-ray done when I was feeling a pain in my Ankle. As per custom, I visited my Orthopedic Physician; he did a quick check-up by asking me to stand on my toes, flex my ankle, and some other checks. The Physician felt everything was fine, but as a precaution asked to take an X-ray of my Left ankle.

My Physician did not have any X-Ray machine at his clinic.

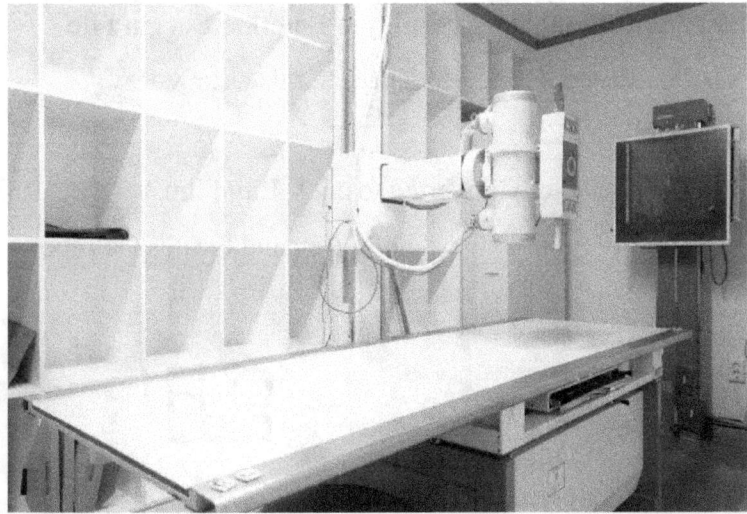

Hence, I visited a nearby Hospital. The first thing which I had to do was go to the Front Desk employee and show them the Physicians prescription. The Front desk Employee took a file and wrote my name along with the test details. She asked me to wait for my name to be called out.

In some cases, you might not get an immediate appointment or given another date. After some time, my name was called out, and I went to a room on the left, which said, "CAUTION X-Ray Radiation." After entering, I was asked to sit up on the table and keep my foot in a specific manner. Once the technician was all set, he put some kind of a Cassette below the table. After some initial research, I understood the Cassette had an X-Ray Detector, and the Cassette itself was a holder. The technician went to another small room to avoid the radiation and took the X-ray. He came back in the room, took the X-Ray Detector, and put the same in some kind of a big box. Once he did that, he was able to view the X-Ray on his Workstation Monitor. This X-Ray is printed and given after some time; this also contains information about the Radiologists interpretation. I showed the same to my Physician, and he mentioned everything seems fine. Now, let us break this information into smaller areas as below;

1. **Imaging Order:** The Physician Prescription
2. **Patient Registration**: Front Desk Employee Entering Data in File
3. **Scheduling Order**: Based on the Modality (In this case X-Ray)
4. **Radiology Exam**: X-Ray Exam.
5. **Conversion**: X-Ray Detector Converted to an X-Ray Film.
6. **Review Report**: Radiologist reviews the X-Ray and creates the report.

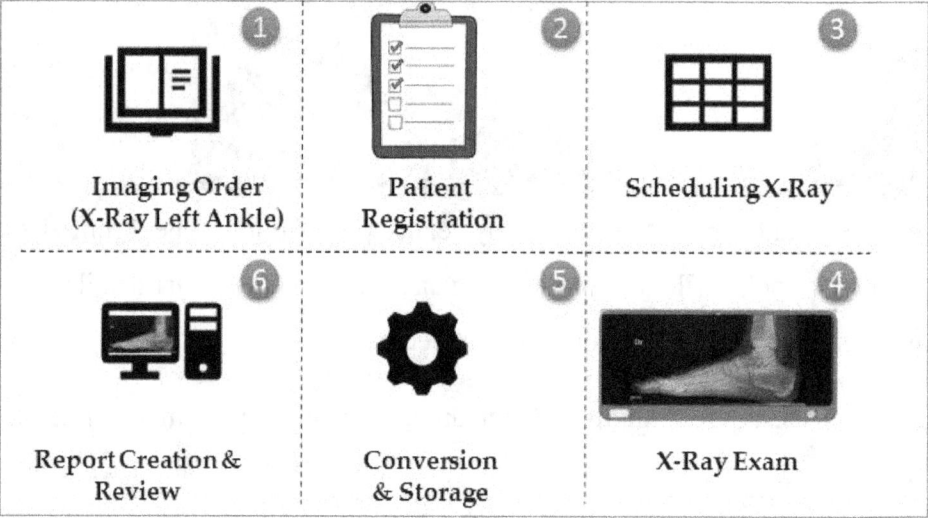

In the overall flow, the last two steps point five and six use DICOM. In simple words, DICOM is a way of sharing Radiology images with different entities. A word document has an extension of ".doc," similarly a DICOM file has the extension of ".dcm". A PACS system stores DICOM images. PACS here stands for Picture Archiving and Communication System.

DICOM was formulated in the 1980s by ACR (American College of Radiology) and NEMA (National Electrical Manufacturers Association). Similar to HL7, CCD, and EDI, DICOM has a specific structure.

We will break down the structure very briefly so that it does not become highly complicated. The DICOM file has four specific sections;

Patient: This section has details around the Patient, Name, Date of Birth, etc.

Study: This section has details of the study done on the Patient, Study Date, Referring Physician.

Series: This section has details around the Modality Type, e.g. RG = Radiographic Imaging (conventional film/screen) as well as the Manufacturer, e.g., Siemens.

Image: This section has details of the Image broken up as Pixels.

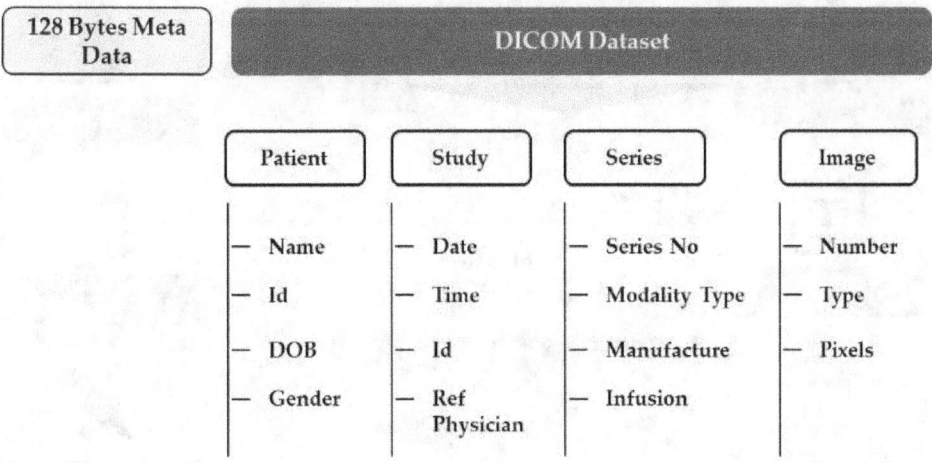

If you follow Kaggle and other Analytics websites, there are various competitions hosted for DICOM images viz: Chest X-Rays, Diabetic Retinopathy. The purpose is to find improved solutions for specific areas using technology. There are many more things which are there in DICOM, but I will stop before things become too complicated ☺.

By the way, one last point before I move to the next topic, did you know that X-Rays were discovered in 1895 by Wilhelm Conrad, Professor at a German University.

7. FHIR:

FHIR is **Fast Healthcare Interoperability Standard,** a standard developed by HL7 for exchanging health information electronically and it is one of the latest formats. That is all I will talk about this specific format ☺

The following workflow shows the standards used at various stages for data transmission:

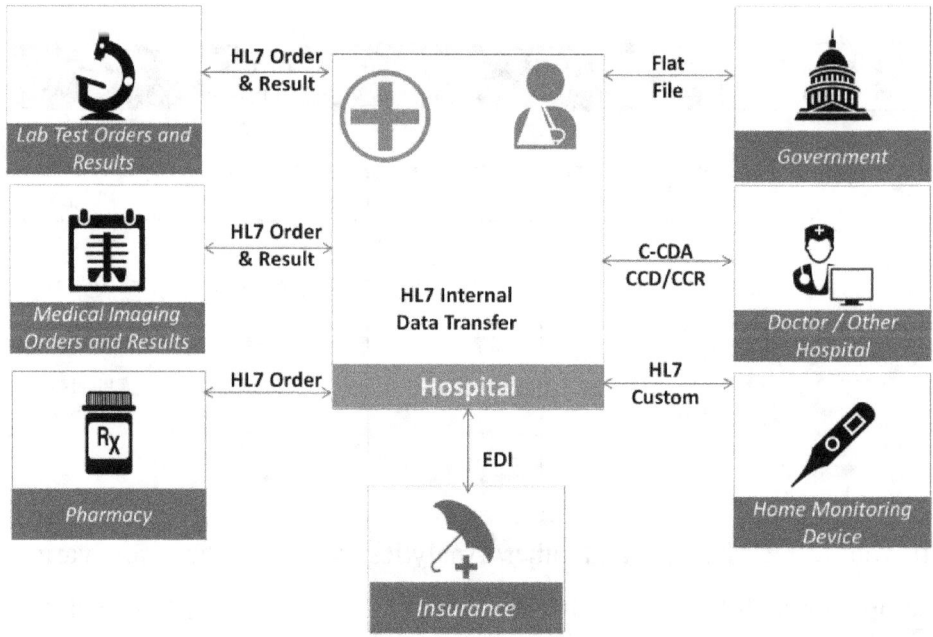

Figure: Healthcare Data Transmission within Stakeholders

#9 What About Coding?

I f you are an IT person, then you must be thinking of what Coding is in Healthcare? Is it Java or.Net? No, it is neither. It is related to Medical Coding, which is converting the Clinical Notes into a Number which can be understood by the Computer. Medical Coders do Medical Coding; these are professionals who understand Medical Terms. The complete Patient Journey generates a lot of Clinical Documentation consisting of Physicians Notes, Nurse Notes, Lab Results, Radiology Results. The Medical Coder will read through all the Clinical Notes and convert specific keywords into Diagnosis Codes. Let us look at an Example

Sample Physician Note:

Chief Complaint: Patient Ross Andrews came to the hospital with Diarrhea for the past three days with Abdominal Pain. Ross had taken Imodium for one day but did not see much of a change.

Diagnosis: The probable diagnosis was Ulcerative colitis

The ICD 9 code for Ulcerative Colitis is K51.90, which is the diagnosis code leveraged for billing calculations.

The below image shows a summary of the steps followed in Medical Coding. Medical Coders would receive Patient-Specific Data, which would include all possible patient information. Patient information includes all possible documentation generated at each step of the patient cycle. After the coder has the files, he/she will do pre-coding (abstraction) which includes parameters like Place of Service, Physician's Name, and any price modifiers. After this, the Coder will Code for Diagnosis and Procedure Codes. Once all Codes are looked up, a peer review will be done and finally an Audit if required. The review is a very important step because any mistake in the Code can result in the Claim being put on hold or even being denied. Finally, the Coded files are used by the Care Provider for Claim generation.

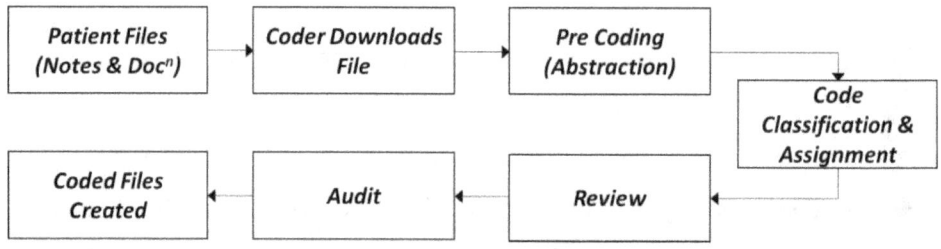

Figure: Medical Coding Workflow

As mentioned earlier, the first references of ICD codes date back to the 1700s, and the main purpose was to record deaths and mortality rate. But in the 1970s, ICD was also expanded to include clinical diagnosis around illness and injuries. ICD-9 has only 13,000 diagnosis codes while ICD-10 has 67,000 Diagnosis Codes.

Let us look at the structure of ICD-9 codes; they are 3-5 digits with the 4th and 5th digit after the decimal. If you notice the first character can be a number, alphabet "E" or alphabet "V." Codes starting with "E" are called "E Code" and are codes for external causes of injury. Codes starting with "V" are called "V Code" and are used to Identify circumstances for encounter related to circumstances other than a disease or injury, e.g., Birth Status for Newborn Babies.

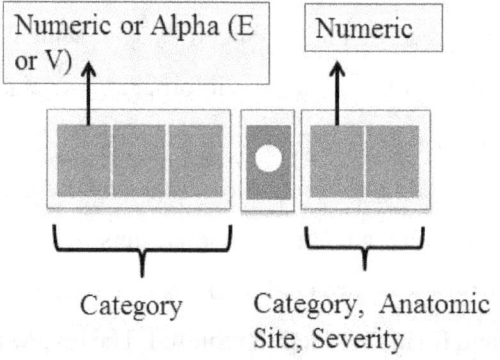

Other Examples of ICD-9 CM codes

- *003.20 = Localized Salmonella Infection, Unspecified*
- *003.21 = Salmonella Meningitis*
- *003.8 = Other specified salmonella infections*
- *003.9 = Salmonella infection, unspecified*
- *V30 Single liveborn*
- *e820–e825 Motor vehicle non-traffic accidents*

Medical coders should Code to the 5th digit wherever possible, which is the highest level of specificity in ICD-9 codes.

Across the world now everyone uses ICD-10, hence it makes sense to understand the structure of ICD-10 as well.

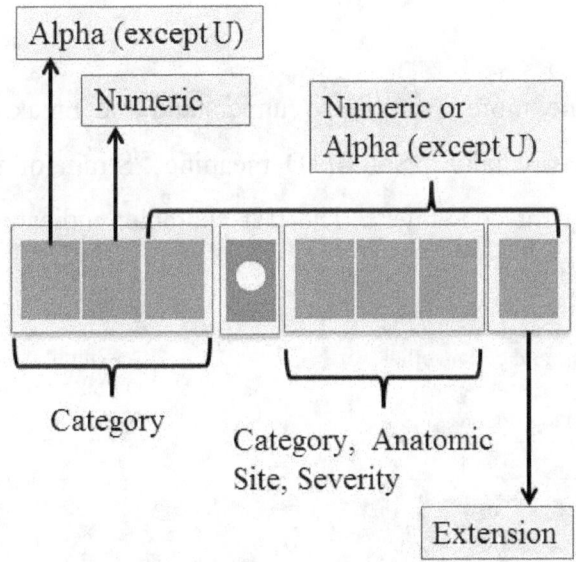

ICD-10 is more complicated when compared to ICD-9. Just look at ICD-10 CM which has 68,000 codes and each code can be anywhere between 3 to 7 characters. ICD-10 provides more flexibility, more detailed, and hence, more specific. If you look at the structure, you will notice each character has a meaning. One of the main benefits of ICD-10 is one can code for laterality. Now, what does Laterality mean? Laterality is identifying left vs. right. In ICD-9 if a patient came with a fracture to the right hand, one could only code for Fracture of the hand as one can't identify right vs. left. In the case of ICD-10, it is easy to code for the same.

Let us take a specific example when making the comparison between ICD-9 and ICD-10

ICD 9 Example

> *813.15: Open Fracture of head of radius*

ICD 10 Example

> *S52123C: Displaced Fracture of head of unspecified radius, initial encounter for open fracture type IIIA, IIIB or IIIC*

Let us take one more example to understand the breakup of ICD-10 characters. We are taking S86.011D meaning "Strain of right Achilles tendon, subsequent encounter". The last character indicates whether the encounter was initial or subsequent.

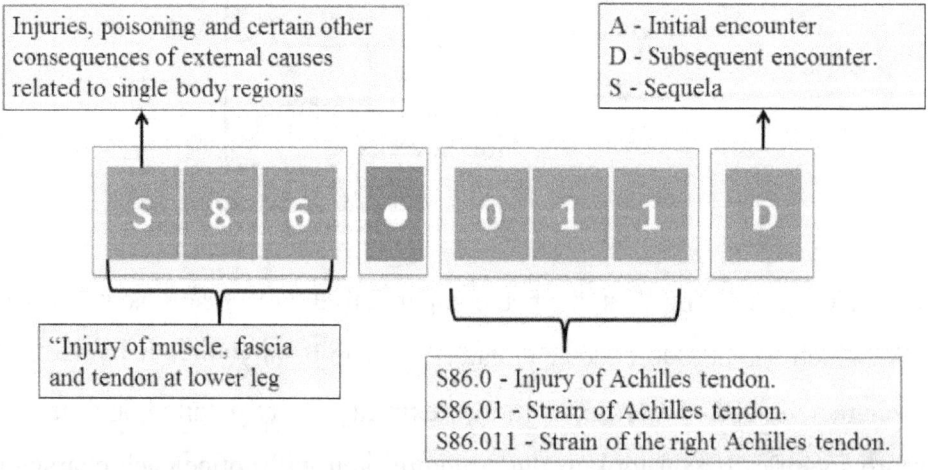

Similarly, we have procedure codes which need coding. ICD 9/10 Procedure codes are primarily for Inpatient reimbursement, and in this case, as well there are ICD-9 and ICD-10 codes. ICD-9 PCS Codes are three to four characters, while ICD-10 PCS are Seven Alphanumeric characters. If you compare the number of codes, it is a huge jump, from approximately 3000 Procedure codes in ICD-9 to 72000 codes in ICD-10. You can imagine the number of new procedures which exist now as compared to earlier. If we look at the below example of the same procedure (Aorta Renal Bypass), we can notice a lot of detail in ICD-10 as compared to ICD-9.

ICD 9 Example

　　　3924: Aorta Renal Bypass

ICD 10 Example

　　　04104J3: Bypass Abdominal Aorta to Right Renal Artery with Synthetic Substitute, Percutaneous Endoscopic Approach

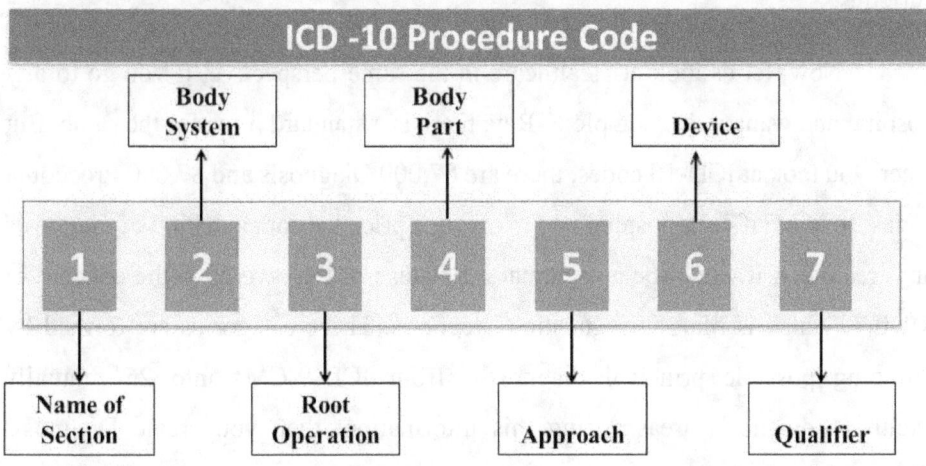

The detail is a benefit of ICD-10, but it also requires more information to be captured as part of clinical documentation. Like in ICD-10 CM (Diagnosis), each character of the code has a meaning. Let us look at another example to make some sense out of the same. I know this is a little complicated but bear with me a little ☺. Let's say the Patient has undergone a knee replacement surgery of the right knee, and we need to code for the same. In ICD-10 the code for knee replacement is "0SRD0JZ" which means Right Knee Joint Replacement. The image explains the meaning of each character, which helps understand in the code R means Replacement, D indicates Right Knee Joint.

But how do I get the billing amount for this Diagnosis code or Procedure Code? Let's take an Analogy to understand some of these numbers/codes. I assume everyone has been to a Retail Store or a Mall for that matter. Each item in the Store which you enter will have a

0	Medical & Surgical Section
S	Lower Joints
R	Replacement
D	Knee Joint, Right
0	Open
J	Synthetic Substitute
Z	No Qualifier

Price Tag on it, so if you want to buy Bread, you will have 5-6 varieties, and each will have a different price. According to your need, you will buy one of the varieties.

Now, let us look at Healthcare in the same perspective, if you go to any hospital and want to do a simple X-Ray, there is a standard price for the same. But when you look at ICD-10 codes, there are 67,000 Diagnosis and 87,000 Procedure codes. Imagine if each hospital had to create a price list for each kind of diagnosis and treatment, it would be a nightmare. Because of this, we have the concept of MDC's, which is Major Diagnostic Categories. These categories are formed by grouping possible principal diagnoses (from ICD-9-CM) into 25 mutually exclusive diagnosis areas. Using this information, then you create Diagnosis Related Groups. Diagnosis-related grouping is formed using MDC's, which help in calculating the possible Amount of treatment for a specific diagnosis. Below is an example of MDC's

MDC	Description
1	Diseases & Disorders of the Nervous System
2	Diseases & Disorders of the Eye
3	Diseases & Disorders of the Ear, Nose, Mouth & Throat
4	Diseases & Disorders of the Respiratory System
5	Diseases & Disorders of the Circulatory System
6	Diseases & Disorders of the Digestive System

One of the most popular DRG systems is MS-DRG, which means Medicare Severity Diagnosis Related Group. Some of the Input parameters given to a DRG software also called as grouper are listed below

a. Patient Diagnosis
b. Procedures performed on the patient
c. Age
d. Gender
e. Discharge Status

Based on these parameters, the software will give a DRG weight, which is one of the O/P parameters. The weight is a payment weight assigned to it based on the average resources used to treat the patient. For example, the DRG weight for a "Coronary Bypass with PTCA w/o MCC" is 5.8183. This weight, when multiplied by the hospital Base Rate, will give the reimbursement amount. The Base Rate is calculated based on the number of discharges, wage and labor rates, and other parameters. If the Base Rate is $5000 then for Coronary Bypass the amount of reimbursement would be 5.8183* $5000 which equals $29091.5

If by chance, due to complications, it took more time/resources to treat a patient, the hospital will need to back it up with documentation. One can also code for the same and there a field called as a Modifier which is present on the claim file. For example, one can Add **Modifier 22** to indicate "Increased Procedural Services." Addition of Modifier 22 can trigger an audit and as mentioned one needs to have Clear Documentation available to support the same viz due to the technical difficulty or the severity of the patient's condition. If Happyville Hospital has a base rate of $6000 and performs the below procedures/treatments, the Reimbursement is equal to Relative Weight multiplied by the Base Rate.

Proc/Condition	Relative Weight	Reimbursement
Lung Transplant	9.3350	$56,010
Simple Pneumonia	0.7096	$4,257
Chronic Obstructive Pulmonary Disease	1.1924	$7,154

The Image on the next page gives an empty UB04 form, which is the Billing form used to send all details to the Insurance company.

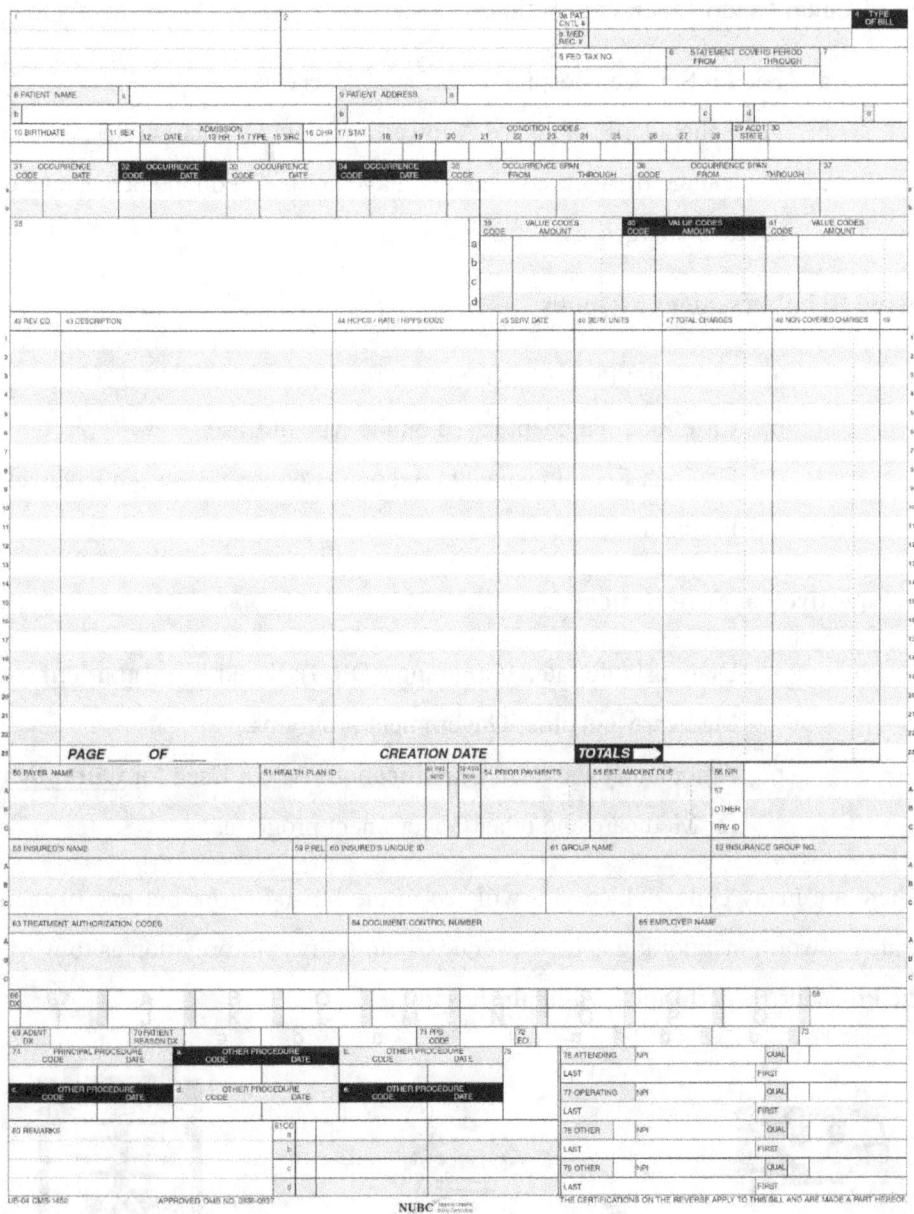

I have not explained many elements in the form, as this book tries to give you a basic understanding of some of the key aspects. By the way, using DRG is just one way of calculating the Reimbursement amount, depending on the type of insurance one can have some of the following methods

Traditional Reimbursement Methods

    a. Fee for Service: Hospital Paid for each service

    b. Fee Schedule: Established Allowed amounts for each service

    c. Percentage of Accrued Charges: Payment based on the percentage of accrued charges

Fixed Reimbursement Methods

    a. Flat Rate: Payment based on a set rate

    b. Case Rate: Payment based on the type of Case

    c. Contract Rate: Payment based on the contract between Payer and Provider.

Prospective Payment System

    a. Diagnosis Related Grouping (DRG): Used for **Inpatient** for Medicare and other Government programs

    b. Ambulatory Payment Classification (APC): Used for **Outpatient** for Medicare and other Government programs

There are many codes which you will see in the UB-04 form, but one of them which is worth mentioning is the Revenue Code. It gives information as to where the Procedure is performed within the hospital.

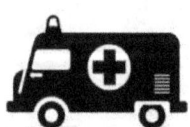

Emergency   **Operating Room**   **Radiology**

The main purpose of the revenue code is to Group similar types of charges onto one line in the Claim form. The table below gives some specific examples for reference.

Revenue Code	Description
11X	Room and Board- Private (Medical or General)
110	General
111	Medical/Surgical/Gyn
25x	Pharmacy
250	General
251	Generic Drugs
29x	Durable Medical Equipment
290	General
291	Rental

#10 My Paper Burden

One way or another, you would have visited a Physician at least once a year. One of the biggest challenges is Data, which you would want to maintain. Let us take the below hypothetical visits and discuss around the same

1. Patient X visits an Eye Physician at least once a year
   a. The Physician will ask some basic questions about the general health of the patient.
   b. The Physician would prescribe some medication if needed
2. Patient X visits a General Physician once every three months
   a. The Physician could ask the patient to do some Lab Tests
   b. Visit a Specialist if required
   c. And again, ask some basic questions would be asked around the general health of the patient
3. Patient X has a fracture and needs to visit an Orthopedist for treatment
   a. The Physician would need to do some X-Ray
   b. Do some Lab Tests to check the basic vitals like CBC etc.
   c. Finally, do surgery if required
4. Finally, Patient X also has an Annual Checkup
   a. The Annual check-up is comprehensive not limited to the below
      i. Many Lab tests like CBC, HbA1c, Serum Glucose, Liver Function Test
      ii. Chest X-Ray

     iii. Full Abdomen Sonography

     iv. Treadmill Test

     v. ECG

  b. The output of the above is a lot of paper documents

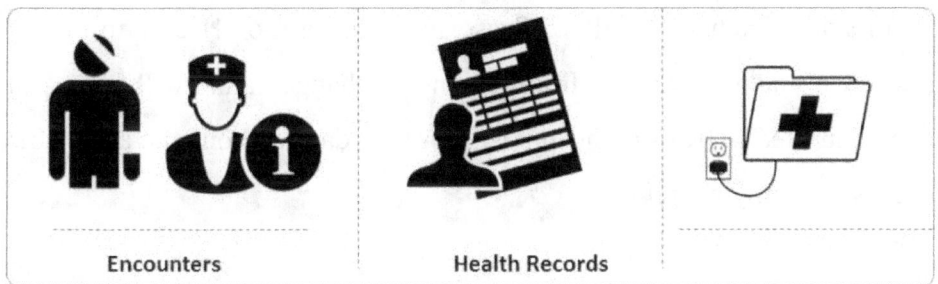

Technically, Patient X is not visiting the same Physician/Hospital/Clinic every time. It is a different physician every time. Imagine the challenge if Patient X is Out for a vacation and faces some problems and visits a Physician. Patient X must explain all his patient history all again because it is not possible to carry so many Paper documents. Most of the Patient Data is at home rather than the hospital, and a Physician would not have access to a lot of this data. To solve this problem, we have the concept of Patient Health Record/Patient Portal. It is like an online Portal which you can access anywhere and anytime. Hospitals and many governments have been promoting the same for some time. But the biggest challenge is User acceptance of using a Portal. It is not like a Bank Account where one login's and checks one's Bank Balance ☺; it's a different concept altogether. I wouldn't want to check my Lab Result every time I log in, would you? But if someone is a Chronic Care Patient, one would want to leverage a Patient Portal or a Chronic Care App to monitor their progress.

Google launched its own Patient Portal but had to shut it down due to lack of user; even Microsoft HealthVault is planning to shut down by the end of

2019. There are even a lot of hospital supported Portals and Mobile Apps, and those would probably work better but would require a lot more push from the Hospital side.

Another Solution which has picked up some steam is the concept of Health Information Exchange (HIE). Please note this is not Health Insurance Exchange rather Health Information Exchange and will like an interconnected EHR of all hospitals. Here, the data will only be accessible to those whom you approve.

#11 This Is everyone Responsibility

Over the years, many wars have been fought worldwide, I don't have any number to quote, but the number could be huge considering world history. One of the greatest military leaders around the 1800's was Napoleon Bonaparte. He was a French Military Leader and fought many wars and conquered most of Europe, though he ultimately was defeated at Waterloo which is the Netherlands in the present day. You might be thinking, "Why Is this guy talking about history," but I will come to my point soon.

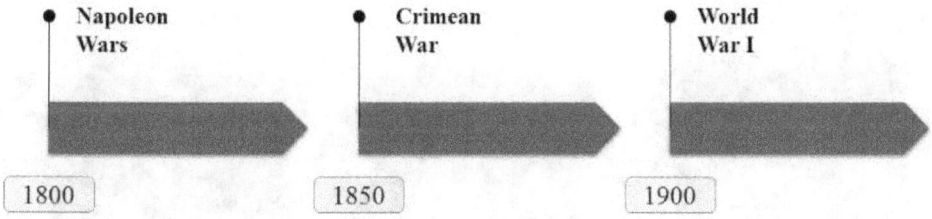

Napoleonic wars ended in the early 1800s; there was also a war in the 1850s fought between Russia and the alliance of Britain, France, Turkey, and Sardinia. The war took place in the Crimean Peninsula, and most deaths happened not due to the war, but due to **typhus, typhoid, cholera, and dysentery**. Britain sent a group of 38 nurses to help their troops in the war, and one of these nurses was Florence Nightingale. The troops wounded in the war were sent to medical stations across the black sea via ships. Nightingale made changes in the sanitation as the entire area was filthy with rats, lice, and fleas. The hospital did not even have clean linen, no soaps. There were even horses which were present in the basement of the hospital, which needed relocation. She made a lot of changes in the sanitation and did a lot of documentation in terms of Hospital Quality. Some of the changes which Nightingale made are listed below

a. Reduce Overcrowding

b. Proper Ventilation

c. Disinfecting the Latrines and drains

Though Nightingale was a Nurse she very meticulous, she used Coxcombs to represent data, and these are now as we know it a variation of Pie Charts. The below image gives an example of the report on Mortality causes during her time in the Crimean War.

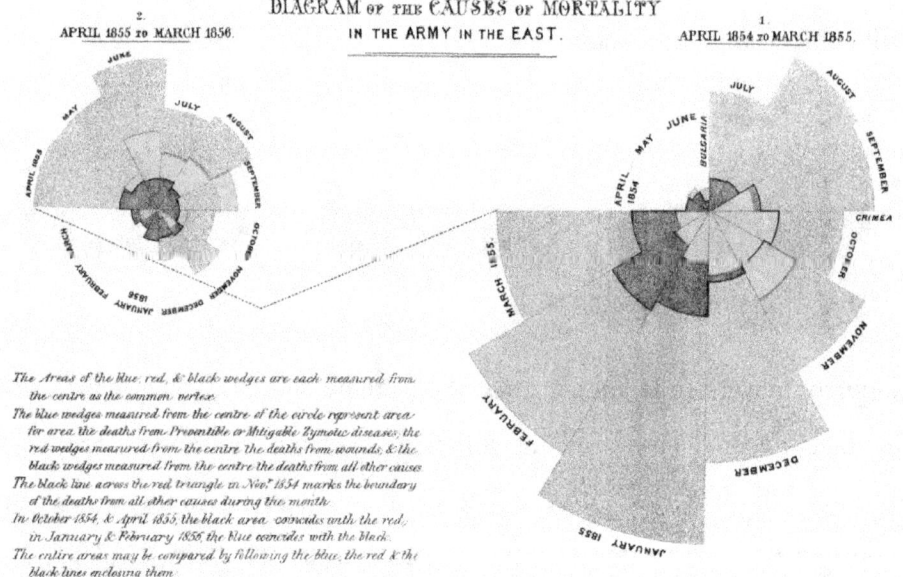

In the year 1860's Louis Pasteur, a French scientist, tried to establish a link between disease and micro-organisms. He conducted many formal experiments to establish this relationship. Did you know that the world knew the existence of germs 200 years before this in 1677? Antoni van

Leeuwenhoek, a Dutch scientist who built a microscope which had pretty good magnification. He saw some tiny organisms in water droplets, which he called "animalcules." Scientists later found these germs in the blood of people and thought the disease caused them. It was only in the 1860s was a relationship established that the germs cause the disease and not the other way around. It was due to this hospital started to follow Sterilization and antiseptic practices.

Other entities also made an impact on how we improve the quality of Healthcare in a hospital. One of them being Dr. Ernest Amory Codman, who used to keep track of patients using "End Results Cards." These cards contained

- Patient Demographics
- Diagnoses
- Treatments
- Outcomes

In 1913 Dr. Codman cofounded American College of Surgeons (ACS) along with Dr. Edward Martin (gynecologist). He started his program to establish certain minimum standards for hospitals. Some of the points included in this are

a. Licensed Physician & Surgeons
b. Rules & Regulations: Regular Staff Meetings for Clinical Reviews.
c. Keeping Medical Records of Patients which included
    - History
    - Lab Results
    - Physical Examination

By the year 1952 Joint Commission on Accreditation of Healthcare Organizations (JCAHO) was formed. The following entities formed it

- American College of Surgeons
- American College of Physicians
- American Hospital Association
- American Medical Association
- Canadian Medical Association

In 1966, Avedis Donabedian, also known as the father of quality assurance, suggested a set of concepts to "Evaluate the Quality of Medical Care." The Paper focuses on one of the facts as to what does "Quality of Medical Care" mean, this can change from organization to another, but it would underlying be dependent on the Goals and Values the Care Organization carries. The Paper mentions many areas and is very comprehensive; a couple of them are mentioned below.

- Approaches to Assessment: What to Assess
  - o The main areas which one can measure
    - Examine the Process of Care
    - **Outcomes** – viz: Surgical fatality rates
- Sources and Methods of Obtaining Information
    - Primarily all research is based on data of Clinical records

It was only in the late 1980s did JHACO implemented a rigorous set of accreditation standards which very much reflected the thoughts of Avedis. As of now, JCAHO accredits and certifies nearly 21,000 health care organizations and programs in the United States. JCAHO standards are the

"Basic Safety Standards," if any Hospital does not pass this, then you might want to reconsider visiting that hospital.

In 1979 NCQA: National Committee for Quality Assurance was formed to review HMO and PPO organizations and at a healthcare provider level. NCQA has worked with various entities to create a set of performance measurement known as HEDIS (Health Plan Employer Data and Information Set) which covers various aspects such as

1. Effectiveness of Care
2. Access and availability of care
3. Cost of Care

Other than accreditation there are other measures also which have come along the way

a. PQRS: Physician Quality Reporting System
   PQRS is a Healthcare Quality Improvement Incentive based Initiative which is driven by CMS (Center for Medicare and Medicaid Services)
   Example: Diabetes: Hemoglobin A1c (HbA1c) Poor Control (>9%)
   Percentage of patients 18-75 years of age with diabetes who had hemoglobin A1c > 9.0% during the measurement period
b. Clinical Quality Measures
   i. These are also part of Meaningful Use which needs to be part of EMR systems
   ii. Example:
      1. Median Time from ED Arrival to ED Departure for Discharged ED Patients

2. Discharged on antithrombotic therapy. Percentage of patients with ischemic stroke given antithrombotic therapy on discharge.

c. ACO Measures

   i. These are measures like Clinical Quality and some related to Patient Safety, Patient Experience

  ii. Example

      1. *Getting Timely Care, Appointments, and Information*

      2. *Patients' Rating of Physician*

      3. *Adult Weight Screening and Follow-up*

#12 Is My Data Secure?

O ne of the most common questions, especially while storing data online, is my data safe? There are many cases of hacking and viruses which happen in the world. After the advent of the internet and especially after 1990, when hospitals started to use Electronic Medical Records, security was a key concern. In 1996 the Healthcare Insurance Portability and Accountability Act (HIPAA) was signed into law. HIPAA primarily covers three areas

- Insurance Portability – this covers the use of EDI for data transmission
- Reduce Fraud and Abuse
- Guarantee Security and Privacy

Who is Covered?

HIPAA is directly applicable to Hospitals, Hospital Employees, Insurance Plans, and Clearinghouses. The reason being these are organizations have direct access to the Healthcare system. But now there is also indirect applicability of HIPAA on organizations/entities which exchange data with those directly covered. This indirect applicability covers Business Associates, Information Technology employees (IT) and to any Outsourced organization. Organizations nowadays, dealing with healthcare data must sign specific HIPAA agreements (HITECH) while individuals are made to sign Business Associate Agreements so that they are legally bound and under a Non-Disclosure agreement.

The Privacy Rule

The privacy rule deals with standards and rules to safeguard/protect the medical condition of an individual. In simple words, you wouldn't want to publicize your bank balance similarly; one also does not like to publicize one's lab results and wouldn't want anyone else to do the same. The Privacy rule deals with one main element known as PHI, known as Protected Health Information. In simple terms, PHI is any information past, present or future which can be used to identify a Patient, the patient's health, or any payment information which might be there. As per HIPAA rules information which can be used to identify a patient should be de-identified or masked or removed from the data before sending to a third party. There are various data elements which qualify as PHI – some of them are listed below

- Name of Patient
- Email Address
- Specific Dates – Date of Birth, Admission Date
- Medical Record Number
- Health Plan Number

Transparency:

HIPAA mandates to provide an accounting of all disclosures of health information. Some of the means are mentioned below

1. Privacy Practice Notice: This requires Payers and Providers to distribute a notice which clearly explains Individual Rights concerning their Health Information
2. If any person asks for the details of the notice, it must be provided by the Payer or Provider or any Covered Entity.

3. The image gives a sample of the notice which each covered must put up either on their website and in their premise.

ZNVille Notice of Privacy Practices

THIS NOTICE DESCRIBES HOW MEDICAL INFORMATION ABOUT YOU MAY BE USED AND DISCLOSED AND HOW YOU CAN GET ACCESS TO THIS INFORMATION. PLEASE REVIEW IT CAREFULLY.

I. General Practice Covered by this Notice

This Notice describes the privacy practices of ZNVille ("General Practice"). "We" and "our" means the General Practice. "You" and "your" means our patient.

II. How to Contact Us/Our Privacy Official

If you have any questions or would like further information about this Notice, you can contact ZNVille's Privacy Official at:

909-909-909

ZNVille

Nashville, TN, 292929

ZNVille@anywhere.com

III. Our Promise to You and Our Legal Obligations

The privacy of your health information is important to us. We understand that your health information is personal, and we are committed to protecting it. This Notice describes how we may use and disclose your protected health information to carry out treatment, payment or health care operations and for other purposes that are permitted or required by law. It also describes your rights to access and control your protected health information. Protected health information is information about you, including demographic information, that may identify you and that relates to your past, present or future physical or mental health or condition and related health care services.

We are required by law to:

- Maintain the privacy of your protected health information;

- Give you this Notice of our legal duties and privacy practices with respect to that information; and

- Abide by the terms of our Notice that is currently in effect.

IV. Last Revision Date

This Notice was last revised on 01st Jan 2019

V. How We May Use or Disclose Your Health Information

Figure: Sample Privacy Notice

---

4. The notice overall talks about the following areas which cover Uses and Disclosures
   a. **Common Uses and Disclosures**: To whom all is patient information commonly disclosed following is a small list
      i. Treatment
      ii. Payment
      iii. Appointment reminders
      iv. Disclosure to Family & Friends
      v. Disclosure to Business Associates
   b. **Less Common Uses and Disclosures**:
      i. Required by Law: In some cases, health information may have to be shared with the Department of Health and Human Services to investigate complaints
      ii. Lawsuits and Legal Actions: Required by a Court order

Collection:

As per HIPAA, one cannot obtain PHI under "pretenses" for obtaining PHI to sell, transfer, or use it for commercial advantage, personal gains.

Access:

As per HIPAA, end-users should have easy access to their health information data. The thought being a chronic care patient would be able to monitor his progress better if he has access to the data. The data can be in the form of "Designated Record Sets," e.g., Electronic Medical Records. As per HHS's website "This includes the right to inspect or obtain a copy, or both, of the PHI, as well as to direct the covered entity to transmit a copy to a designated person or entity of the individual's choice."

Retention:

As per HIPPA, the covered entities must maintain the following information for six years. Some of the documents are below; please note this is not exhaustive just a sample.

- Policies & Procedures implemented to Comply with HIPAA; this is as per CFR §164.316(b)(1) and (2)
- Authorizations received for disclosure of PHI
- Information Security & Privacy Policy
- Incident Notification Documentation
- Internal Audit documents

Security:

This section talks about various standards which need to be implemented, especially in the case of Electronically transmitted data. Some of the rules are listed below

- **Role-Based Access**: Each user accessing patients Medical Record should specific Access. Not all employees would have access to all the patient level information
- **Data Encryption**: This is a method using which data must be encoded using a key and can be read or decoded only using that key. If data is sent to external entities, Data encryption should be used as data will go beyond the firewall of the covered entity.
- **Data Masking**: This is another method of de-identifying data so that the patient's identity is protected. A simple example would be to

replace the Specific numbers of SSN (Social Security Number) with Stars, e.g., The number would look like ***-***-1234.

- **Using EDI Standards**: As per HIPAA, the following transactions should be used to transmit data electronically.

EDI	Transaction Set
EDI 837	Health Care Claim Transaction set
EDI 835	Health Care Claim Payment Transaction Set
EDI 834	Benefit Enrollment and Maintenance Set
EDI 820	Payroll Deducted and other group Premium Payment for Insurance Products
EDI 270	Health Care Eligibility/Benefit Inquiry
EDI 271	Health Care Eligibility/Benefit Response
EDI 276	Health Care Claim Status Request
EDI 277	Health Care Claim Status Notification
EDI 278	Health Care Service Review Information
EDI 997	Functional Acknowledgement Transaction Set

Accuracy & Correction:

As per HIPAA if the patient finds an error in his/her medical record, one has the right to get the same amended. Following is a small excerpt from CFR §164.526

"Individual has the right to have a covered entity amend protected health information or a record about the individual in a designated record set."

Medical Records are legal records, and to make corrections, one needs to make amendments to the same. As per the amendment received, the data should be amended within 60 days. The output of the same can be any of the two

- **Acceptance**: If the covered entity agrees with your request, you will receive an acceptance, and there will be an amendment.
- **Denial**: If the covered entity disagrees with your request, you will receive a written denial, and there won't be an amendment. The written denial would include the reason for denial.

Penalty:

Since HIPAA is a law dealing with very sensitive Patient Information, breaking the law will attract penalties. These penalties can range from anywhere between $100 to $50,000 per violation. The max penalty for a year is $1.5 million, and there can also be criminal penalties.

To understand all of the above little bit more, let us look at some real-life examples.

Privacy Violation Example:

I am not sure if you have heard of the case of Huping Zhou which occurred in April of 2010. Mr. Huping was a former researcher at the UCLA Healthcare System. Huping has accessed Medical records of his co-workers and many celebrities / high profile individuals. He did this not One or two times but over three hundred times. As per the cbsnews he accessed Medical Records (without any specific reason) of celebs like Tom Hanks, Leonardo DiCaprio, Drew Barrymore. Huping was sentenced to four months in prison with a fine of $2000/-

Transparency Issues:

Do you use Social Media? I assume, yes. The reason I ask is that many times we create an ID on a website need not be social media but also for buying stuff. We normally don't read what comes as a pop-up we go on clicking Yes/Next/Proceed. One of those pages has details of the Privacy and Security agreement of that site and how your data will be used. Ideally, your data is not supposed to be sold to anyone else if it is then that is an issue. You might have heard the news of Cambridge Analytica that is a violation of privacy as well as transparency. Similarly, in the case of Healthcare, there are a lot of mobile Apps which have come up in the market, viz: For Chronic Care Monitoring. As per a study conducted by BMJ, 79% of the Apps (Study was done on 24 Apps) lacked transparency as to how the data was going to be used.

Access Issues:

If you leave an Organization, do you still have access to the systems of that Organization? If the Answer is yes, then that is a big problem! Normally this should not happen as once an employee leaves, his access gets purged/removed. This is not what happened with Colorado-based Pagosa Springs Medical Center. The office for civil rights received a complaint that a Former employee of the Colorado hospital still had access to the web-based scheduling calendar. On further investigation, it was found that the employee had accessed the calendar on two occasions in July and September of 2013. The calendar had electronically protected the health information of 500+ patients. Due to the failure of not terminating the access of the former employee, the Colorado hospital was penalized for $111,400.

#13 Continuous Improvement –

Reporting & Analytics

The banking industry has been around for long, and if you look at the IT side, there too, there has been a lot of automation on the Banking side. Let's take a simple example, once I used my debit card multiple times in a span of say around ten minutes with the total amount being substantially high. One more thing, I used my debit card at different shops. As soon I was done, I got a call from the bank; asking me, "Did you make if multiple transactions from your debit card."

Imagine if the same could happen in healthcare but only that the actors are different viz the patient and the Physician. Chronic care patients could leverage this concept, consider a patient who monitors his sugar and blood pressure regularly.

In terms of analogy, if we replace items bought with items eaten, one can monitor the calorie intake by using a smartphone. The patient monitors and records the following:

- Fasting sugar
- Post-lunch sugar
- Breakfast, Lunch, and Dinner

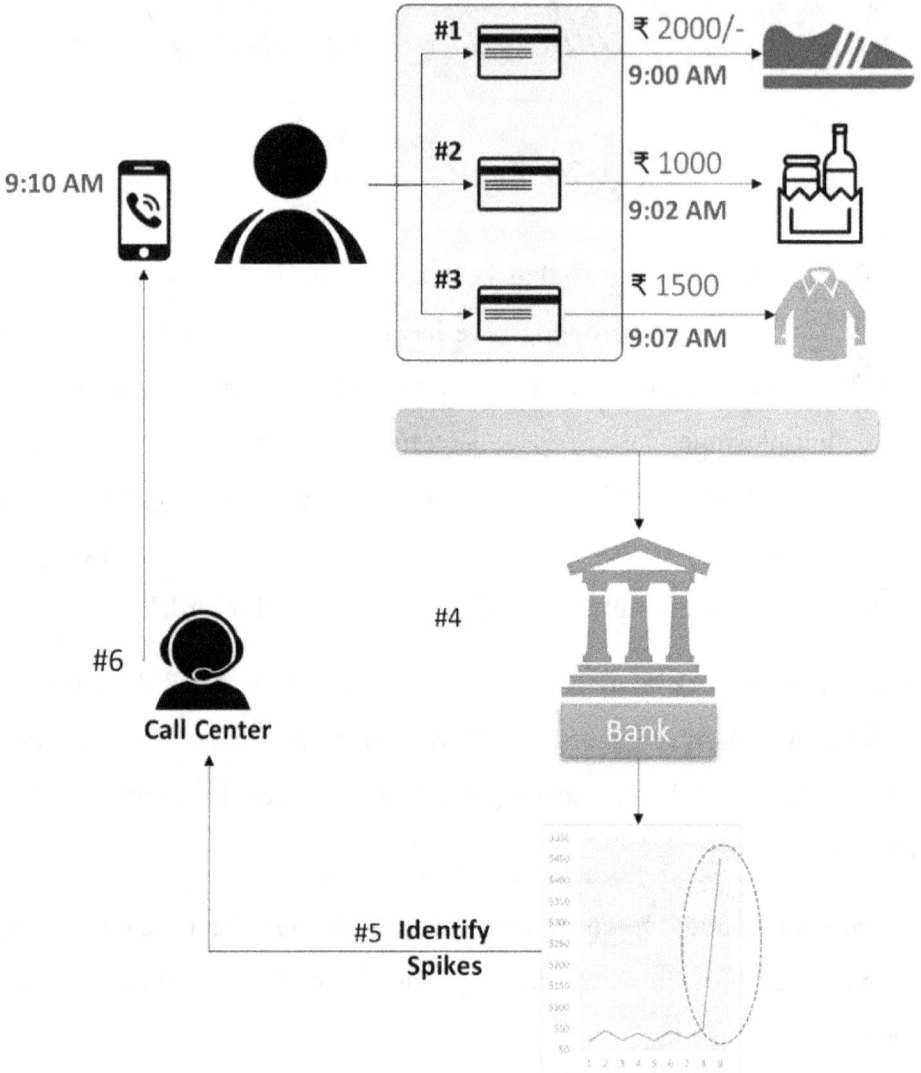

Figure: Banking Example

The patient can also enter the duration of exercise/activities he did during the day. All the data entered by the patient in his smartphone App can integrate with the Hospital Information system. Based on this data and other analysis, the Physician could alert the patient and make some informed decisions.

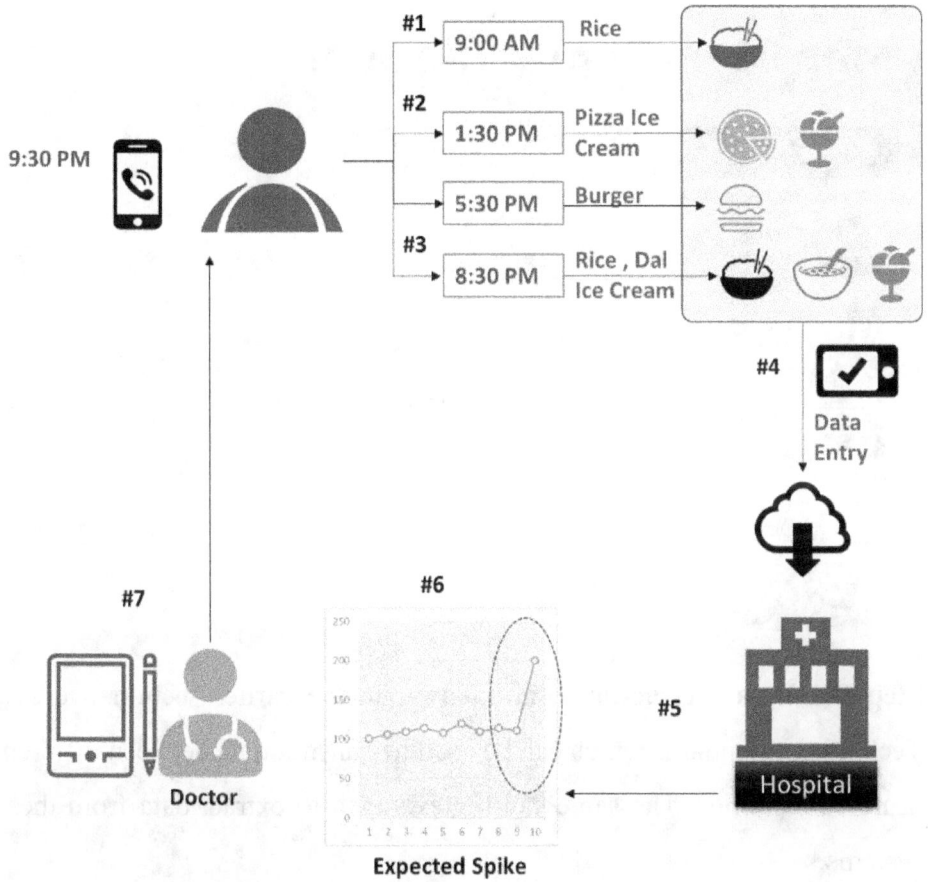

Figure: Healthcare Example

Above example gives an example of a remote patient monitoring system but not so easy to implement since in this case, data needs to be entered by the patient manually. Let us now detail some of the steps we need to follow when we need to do any reporting and analytics within a hospital.

Before we do any reporting or analytics, we need to follow some of the steps

Step 01: Identify the Source Systems – this piece we saw when we detailed the Revenue cycle system as well as the EMR systems. From a Hospital perspective, we understood the possible source systems.

Step 01 – Identify The Sources

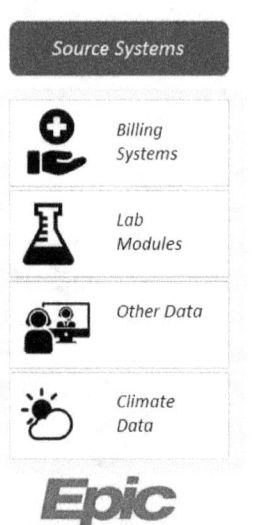

Step 02: Data Extraction Standards – In the earlier section, we saw Technology standards which can be used to transmit data between different healthcare entities. The same can be leveraged to extract data from these systems.

Step 02 – Data Extraction Standards

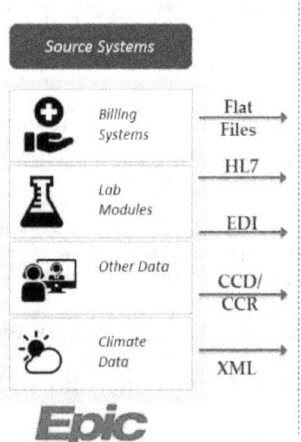

Step 03: Data Cleaning/Quality – This is a very important phase as this step requires a lot of detailed analysis. This step covers many other steps viz, data deduplication, data standardization, data normalization, and others. Let us look at some examples to explain some of these points.

Data Deduplication: A common challenge handling patient information is duplication of data.

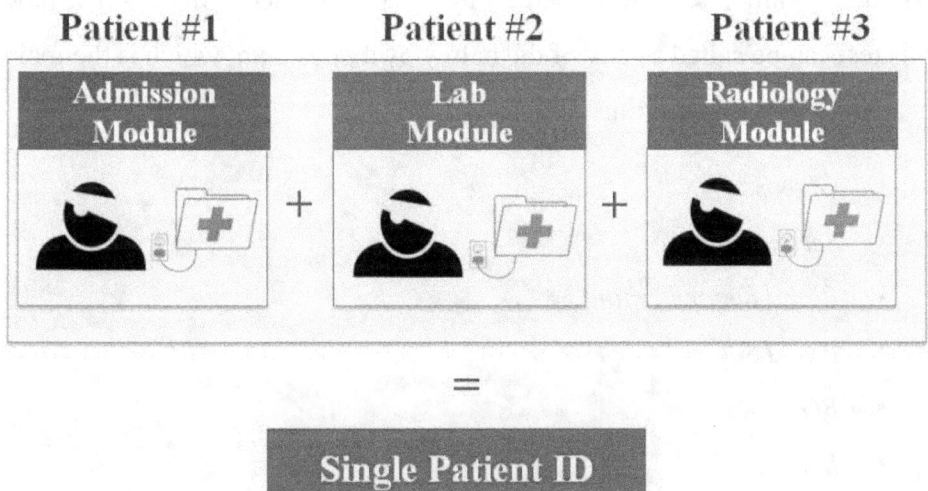

If the Hospital is using different EMR Systems for different modules, then each module can assign a separate ID internally for the same patient. To create a single Patient Id, one would need to match other parameters viz name, age, date of admission, address, SSN, and other elements.

Data Standardization: Let's look at one of the most common blood tests done in a hospital – Common Blood Count (CBC), which gives a lot of parameters, including Hemoglobin. The normal value of Hemoglobin for Men should be between 13.8 to 17.2 (g/dL), and for Women, it is between 12.1 to 15.1 g/dL. Everything looks simple till now but look at the unit of measurement g/dL; the value can be any of the following, which is the challenge.

- grams per deciliter (g/dL)
- grams per liter (g/L)
- milligrams per liter (g/L)
- milligrams per deciliter (mg/dL)

Another common test prescribed a Physician is to check Blood Sugar now this test can be called as any of the below by a physician, which is the main challenge for standardizing clinical data.

- *Glucose*
- *Serum Glucose*
- *Blood Sugar Fasting*
- *Blood Sugar*
- *BG*
- *BGL*
- *BSL*

A tool used by many for some of the standardization is Relma.

Step 03 – Data Cleaning

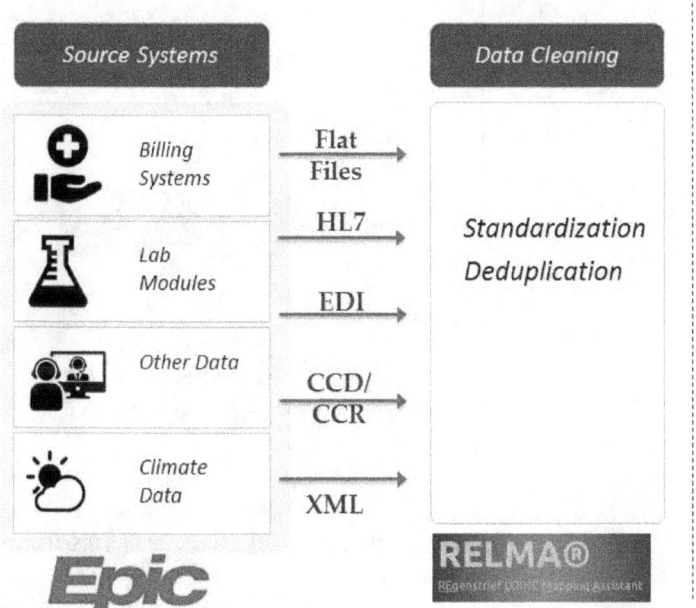

Step 04 Logical Data Model: This is the step where we create a Logical Database. In simple terms, we create a list of data elements which are stored in each entity. Example Patient Master would contain elements like Patient Name, Date of Birth. The Model gives an example of how all tables relate to each other. The below Figure gives an example of a Simple Data Model.

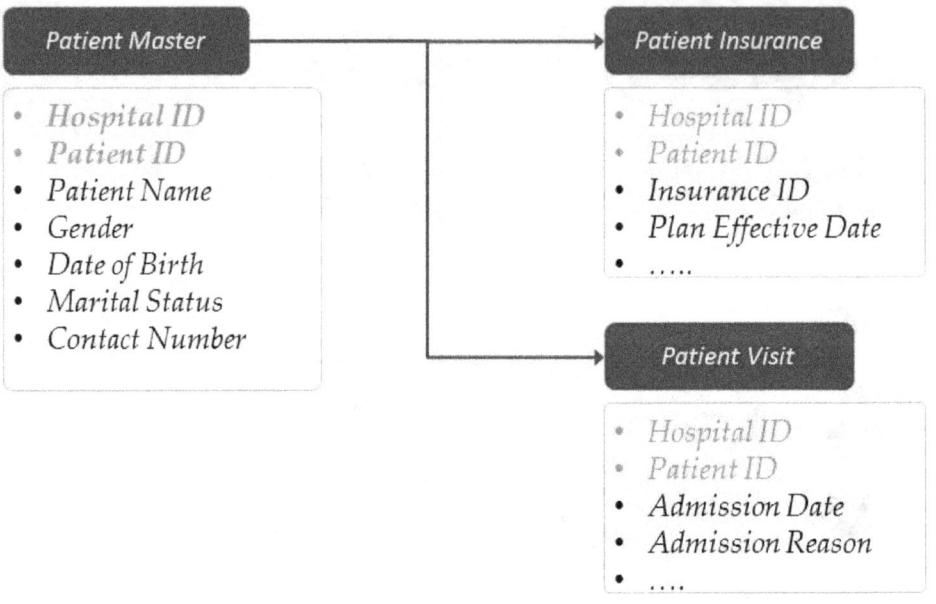

There are many tools used by organizations viz: SQL Server, MySql, and others for this.

Step 04 – Logical Data Model

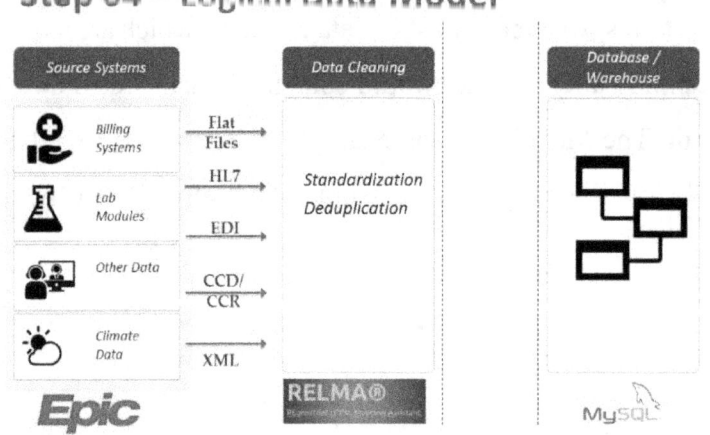

Step 05 Load the Data: The next step is to copy the data in the data warehouse viz the standardized/cleansed data, which we will use for reporting. At this stage, we can use many tools in the market like Informatica, DMExpress, SSIS. One of the common tools used in healthcare

is Mirth, which is an Enterprise Integration Engine customized for healthcare as it is capable of easily understanding Healthcare Standards Viz HL7, EDI.

Step 05 – Load the Data

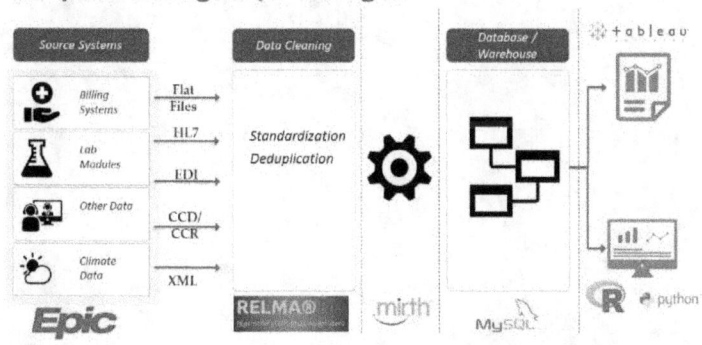

Step 06 Insights or Foresights: Once we have all the data in the data warehouse, we can now analyze the data as we wish. There are two ways in which one can analyze the data – Insights or Foresights.

Step 06 – Insights / Foresight

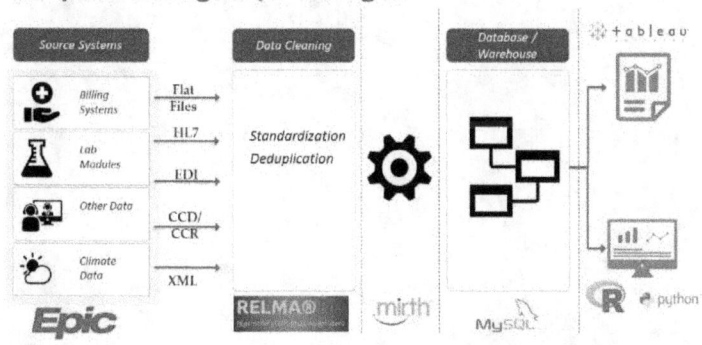

Insights mean analyzing what has already happened, i.e., visually showcasing data of what has already happened. Visualization can be done using Tools like Tableau, PowerBI, or any other Reporting Tool.

Foresight is analyzing the data of the past and showcasing what can happen in the future; which is done using Forecasting, Machine Learning, Deep Learning using tools like R Programming and Python. The output of this can be again visually representing using Tableau or any other Reporting tool.

Some sample KPIs are listed below

- Insight Examples:
  - Total number of Inpatients visiting the hospital Monthly
  - Number of Readmissions
  - Number of Claim Denials
  - Month on Month Revenue Analysis
- Foresight Examples
  - Forecast Patient Volume for Coming month
  - Find the Probability of Patient Readmission
  - Identify High-Risk Patients (disease-specific)

#14 What's New?

Internet of Things

Kevin Ashton phrased the term Internet of Things in 1999, but IoT has been around for much before, i.e., the 1990s. Gartner mentions the number of connected things would touch near to 20 billion. IoT has always focused on Smart Homes, and there are many supporting scenarios. You might have heard/read the example of a company which offered their employees to get a microchip embedded in their hands. The employees could use which employees could enter the office, log on to their PC. By the way, the companies name is Three Square Market, and the story is of August 2017.

We have seen a growing trend around Smartwatches using which one can track basic information like heart rate, no of steps taken. The Smartwatch has a sensor/actuator to gather this information and can interface data using Bluetooth or Wi-Fi. This data can interface with various systems like Patient Portals, Hospital Systems.

Every year around my birth month, my office sends me for an annual health checkup, to set up an appointment, I log in to my Office's HRMS system and schedule a specific date. Other than my annual checkup if I am not feeling well and I want to go to the hospital, either I will call up and schedule an appointment or just walk-in to the clinic. Now, if a chronic care patient is unwell, he will also do the same, i.e., schedule an appointment or walk-in. But, with an increase in Home Health, using IoT Physicians can monitor

Patients Vitals and other parameters easily. One can also create a mechanism to automatically schedule an Appointment if specific Monitoring Parameters don't seem correct. Would we want to do this for everyone? I don't believe it would make sense; it will help to limit this volume to a specific set of patients (e.g., Chronic Care Patients). Once I reach the clinic for my annual checkup, the front desk employee asks for some documentation; I don't have to fill in many details as the clinic has some of my basic information.

Many times, I think, how does a hospital get information about a critical person (Casualty), especially if no one is with the patient. One possible solution to this problem could be biometric sensors, using which one could get Basic Information of the Patient, this, in turn, will save time and improve Patient Satisfaction. The sensors would be possible in places where Governments/Organizations have already bio-metric Id's, e.g., India using Aadhar.

Some Hospitals at the time of registration give the patient an RFID Tag (I did not get one), with the help of which the hospital can track the patient movement. A good example is that of Apollo Hospitals in Chennai; they use ICEGEN's "Patient Mantra" Solution, which helps them Locate and Track each Patient. Due to this, the Hospital was able to easily track patients who were going through 26 diagnostic procedures in one day. They were also able to identify which area is getting crowded and thus make some corrections.

Insurance Eligibility is not only one of the most crucial steps in the Patient Journey but also many times the most complex. Since mine was an annual checkup sponsored by my company, I did not need to provide any insurance details. At this point, there isn't any sensor which can check the insurance eligibility of a person; solutions like pokitdok provide a Cloud-based API to validate Insurance and can help improve the efficiency of the process.

In my annual check-up, the first step I had to do was give my blood sample, and I had to wait for my turn. The Lab technician follows a standard procedure while drawing blood; one important aspect I notice at this time I notice is keeping the environment clean. Before drawing blood, he used a hand sanitizer, wore a new set of Gloves, and opened a new set of Syringe and needles. At the end of the process, the technician throws the syringe and needle in a bin labeled as bio-waste.

Cleanliness is very crucial for a Care Provider, as approximately 10% of Total Healthcare costs are due to Healthcare Associated Infection or Hospital Acquired Infection (HAI). Statistics show that more people die of HAI each year as compared to Breast Cancer and Prostate Cancer combined. Ohio Health uses RFID to track Hand-Hygiene Health Compliance to try and keep HAI in check. Before visiting a Patient, a Physician needs to wash their hands, Ohio Health installed RFID sensors at washing stations to check if Physicians visited the washing station and based on statistics captured physicians are given feedback.

In case a Patient needs to be admitted, it is important to clean and ready the room for the patient. IoT in this space has done wonders for some hospitals. Bed Side Sensors at a New York Hospital help them to find out Bed Availability. Temperature Sensors monitor the Temperature of the Room before the patient enters the room. Hospitals in the UK have combined the use of RFIDs/Sensors and Prediction Models to check when a Bed could become available and thus improve efficiency.

After giving my blood sample, I was asked to wait in a room for my Stress test (running on a Treadmill). As a setup procedure, I was made to wear a small device with leads connected to my chest. The small device was in turn connected was to a machine (on a trolley) with a small display which was showing my vitals. Before the procedure starts (i.e., I am told to run on the treadmill) the Physician took my Blood Pressure, and as the procedure starts, the Physician keeps measuring my BP 2-3 times. Once the procedure completes, the Physician measures my BP one final time. All the time, the Physician keeps entering this data in the system.

Like this device/machine, the hospital has various other Point of Care Sensors/devices like Pulse Oximeter, ECG, Electromyogram, Body Position other than the standard Blood Pressure Monitor, Glucometer. Various Hospitals have built interfaces with these devices/sensors to capture this data in their HIS/EMR Systems automatically. By doing, so Hospitals gets benefits of reduced errors due to Data Entry and real-time monitoring of patients. A Hospital in Bengaluru (India) uses a wearable Fetal Monitoring device for expecting mothers, which are integrated with a Mobile App and the Hospitals Information System. The App showcases information such as fetal heart rate, and the Physician can monitor the same to take real-time decisions. Apollo Hospitals in Chennai has connected all Medical Equipment to its Hospital Information System and doing so helps to monitor patients via a centralized system.

Another aspect to note here was documentation done by the Lab Technician, Nurse, and Physicians. This documentation is a crucial phase one to treat a patient and for billing purposes, as this data is used by Medical Coders to enter the ICD Codes. There are tools in the market which can help Physicians improve productivity, one example being of Nuance - Intelligent

Virtual Assistant – Florence launched in 2015. Florence is a combination of IoT and Artificial Intelligence and has various voice-driven workflows using which Physicians can capture vitals as well as place orders.

In the beginning, we talked about how hospitals use RFID's to track patients. Do you think hospitals could use RFID's to track equipment's? Yes, they do, and one of the top reasons to do so is Theft!!! I heard of thieves breaking in a bank, but could not believe that could happen in a hospital? Thieves come dressed as employees and steal medical equipment. Hospitals use IoT (RFID) to help track various aspects of medical equipment like location, temperature, usage, and electricity consumption in some cases. By doing so, Hospitals can monitor thefts, but this can also help reduce the cost of maintenance and improve patient satisfaction.

At the end of the check-up, the data of all the Patient interactions would be sent to the billing team for billing and claim filing. IoT might not have a direct role in most of the Back-office processes, but there are some processes which could benefit by using IoT like Billing. We talked about Patients being given RFID Tags at the time of registration, which can also be used to track and locate a patient. The same RFID Tag can help track the duration a patient is at a specific department; this can be used for Emergency Patients. In some cases, since we track the usage of Medical Equipment, we can use the information to enter the charges in the System.

Where do we go from here?

Overall, we see that IoT in a hospital environment is a growing reality, having said that there are still many challenges while implementing IoT. Security is one of the Top Concerns for IoT as one needs to maintain data privacy and integrity when transmitting data over a network. It becomes even more complex in a healthcare environment where we have HIPAA and other Data Privacy Norms. Another aspect is the lack of common Standards. As IoT is well hardware dependent, and there are so many diverse types of equipment's/devices, each having a different method of communication. This makes it complicated and time-consuming to build interfaces with Hospital Systems (EMR) to capture the data electronically.

Telemedicine: The 100-Year-Old Prediction

Do you like visiting a hospital? I am not sure many people like to do that. It is not like you are visiting a Bank to check your Account Balance, that too can be done online nowadays. Some might even argue we don't like visiting a Bank after 15th of the month, and I am talking about Salaried employees here ☺, but that is a separate discussion altogether.

In many cases, you will visit a hospital when you don't have an option remaining and have tried all possible remedies. When I say remedies, it can range anywhere from asking your neighbor, friends, Grandma, Uncles & Aunts, and whomsoever you feel can help. Finally, when any of these options don't work, you would prefer speaking to a Physician on a call rather than meeting him. Not that we have anything against a Physician, it's just that we don't like Hospitals ☺.

If we look at history (when I say history, I mean a long time back) the

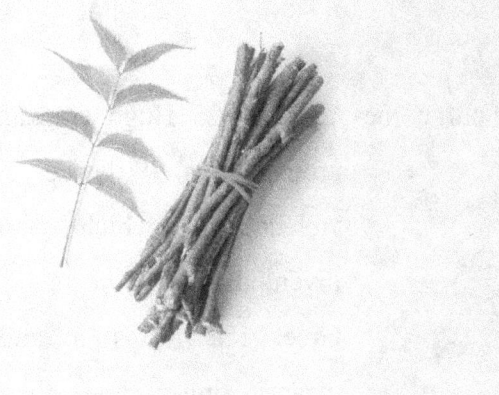

concept of a Hospital did not exist. The Physician/Vaidya used to visit the patient in the comfort of his home for providing treatment. But the situation is completely different now, though few Physicians do come home to provide care most of the care is provided in a Hospital Setting.

Guglielmo Marconi invented the radio in the 1890s, but it was only in the

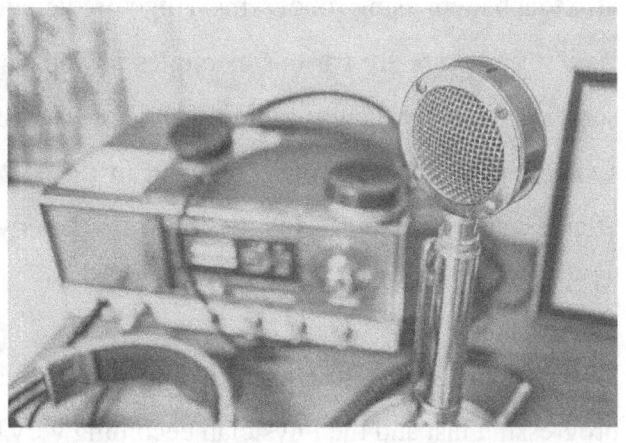

1920s when the radio got the recognition to be a medium of broadcasting information. Hugo Gernsback was one of the few who tried to push the boundaries of technology in the early 1900s. He designed the first home radio set marketed and as Telimco Wireless for $7.50. Hugo also came out with a couple of Tech Magazines (since he was also a publisher) "Modern Electronics" and "Electrical

Experimenter." The second magazine later came to be known as "Science and Invention."

Here is where the interesting part comes, in Feb 1925, Hugo wrote an article 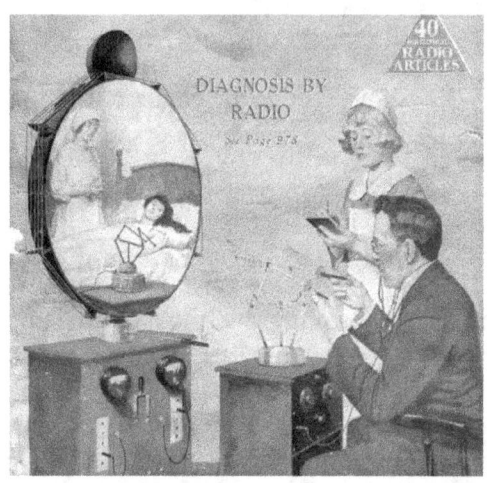 around a device called "teledactyl," which would be invented after 50 years (1975). In Greek, tele means Far, and dactyl means finger and the literal meaning would "feel at a distance." Using this device, a Physician could view the patient through a viewscreen but could also touch them using robot arms. Hugo predicted telemedicine as we know it now, and there are various examples nowadays where surgeons perform surgery remotely using robotic devices. But it is fascinating to note something which was conceptualized in the 1920s has picked up almost after a century in 2000s. Oh, by the way, the cover of the Magazine said, "The Radio Physician–Maybe."

Hugo's logic was also sound in forecasting this, as he saw technology progressing fast and the Physician becoming very busy to make house calls. In the article, he also refers to the changing people mindset, of how instead of visiting friends we call them, (nowadays we don't even call them we WhatsApp them ☺) and instead of visiting a concert we watch television programs (today it is Cable Tv, Netflix, on-demand services).

So, let us try and decipher the components conceptualized by Hugo around telemedicine in the 1920s. He refers to the two key components, and we will try to validate how easy it for anyone to do so.

1.   **The Viewscreen**: When compared to today's world, it would be a simple video call, anyone with a smartphone can easily do that using Skype, WhatsApp, Facetime.

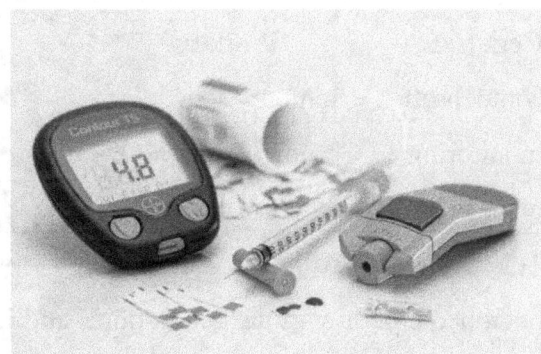

2.   **Get Patient Vitals**: Earlier, you would have to check the pulse manually, but nowadays there are Bluetooth enabled Point of care devices using which one can easily get the patients vitals.

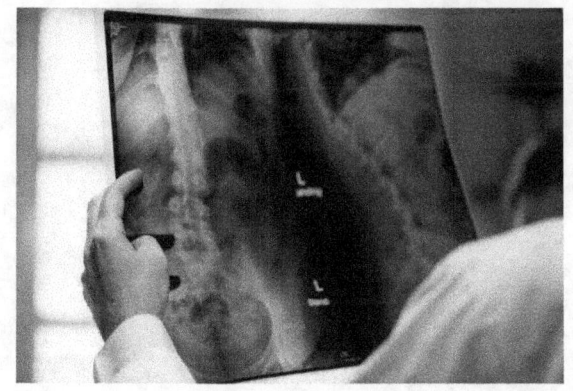

If we look at the current scenario, only these two components will not suffice. I mean there are so many regulations in place, e.g., one needs to be HIPAA compliant; there needs to be detailed clinical documentation for billing. In many cases, the insurance companies do not reimburse telemedicine cases; it is only now that there is a change seen in some areas. Above all, the data also needs to be captured or integrated with EMR systems. One of the first documented use cases of Telemedicine was around teleradiology in the 1950s, wherein radiological images were transmitted over 24 miles using telephone lines. Clinicians at the University of Nebraska first used telemedicine in 1959 for video consultation across the campus. Telemedicine has been growing since then, and various use cases are being implemented for ranging from Rural Health, Geriatrics, Workers compensation, remote ICU monitoring, Chronic care management to Pediatric care. Telemedicine still is an

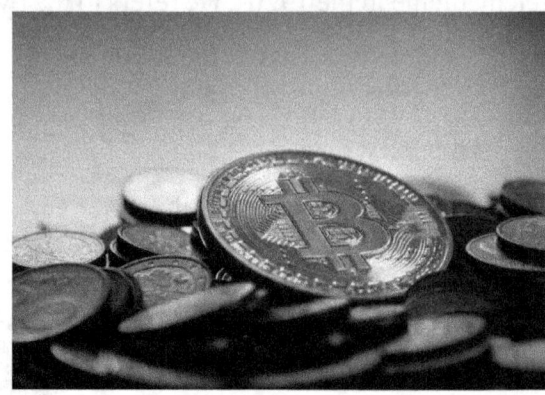

untapped area in various geographies and if you look at its Life is coming full circle from the Physician treating a patient at Home, then in clinics and hospitals and coming back to treating the patient at home but remotely. And by the way, if you search for "teledactyl," you will also find that it is also a blockchain platform being developed specifically for healthcare.

#15 The Hypothetical Billing Example

Let us look at a hypothetical example and try to calculate the amount the Patient would have to pay vs. what the Payer will have to pay. Along the way, we will also try and capture details of data each phase needs to capture.

A Mr. James Brown comes to hospital ZNVille on 2nd January 2013, with a complaint of severe stomachache. Physician Jeremy suspects it to be a case of Food Poisoning and asks Mr. Brown to get admitted so that he can monitor the condition closely. Mrs. Brown had already taken an appointment before meeting the Physician Jeremy. Some of the information which Mrs. Brown at the time is listed below.

Scheduling	
Patient Info	
Name	Mr. James Brown
Age	34
Gender	M
Appointment Date	Wednesday, January 02, 2013
Appointment With	Dr. Jones T.

She was asked for Insurance information as well, and she shared that three insurances and was not sure which one was valid or not. So as part of Pre-registration Insurance details of Humana, Aetna and Cigna were captured.

Pre-Registration	
Patient Info	
Primary Insurance	**Aetna**
Primary Insurance ID	A10020
Secondary Insurance	**Humana**
Secondary Insurance ID	B10020
Tertiary Insurance	**CIGNA**
Tertiary Insurance ID	C10020

The Front desk employee gets the insurance validated. This step is done using an EDI 270/271, which is Insurance Eligibility. At this step, one can get basic things validated viz is the Insurance valid, is the wheelchair covered or is the Ambulance covered? The Payer Response received is as below.

	Payer Response		
	Aetna	**Humana**	**Cigna**
Insurance ID	A10020	B10020	C10020
Insurance Expiry	12/31/2012	12/31/2013	12/31/2013
Insurance Coverage	$10,000	$15,000	$12,000
Coverage Remaining	$2,000	$5,000	$10,000

One can notice that Aetna's Insurance Expired on 12th Dec 2012, while the Patient is admitted on 2nd Jan 2013. Hence, Aetna Insurance cannot be leveraged by Mr. Brown while the other two can be leveraged. Meanwhile, Mrs. Brown is filling the Patient Registration details and enters some of the basic details as below.

Patient Registration	
First Name	James
Last Name	Brown
Gender	M
Date of Birth	1/11/1979
City	New York
Marital Status	Married

Dr. Jeremy starts Mr. Brown on Diphenoxylate 2.5 MG & also orders a Lab Test and some Radiology tests as well. Mr. Brown was treated for three days in the hospital and discharged on the fourth day after lunch, following are some of the data elements which would be captured in the Billing System Day wise.

DAY 01	Description	Code	Revenue Code
Primary Diagnosis	Food Poisoning	ICD 9 - 005.9	
Private General Room			Room and Board- Private 110
Physician Charges			Professional Fees: 988 Consultation
Food Services			Patient Convenience: 991 Cafeteria/Guest Tray
Medication	Diphenoxylate 2.5 MG	RxNorm: 329305	General Drugs: 251

DAY 02	Description	Code	Revenue Code
Order - X-Ray	Abdominal X-Ray	CPT Code: 74010	Radiology Diagnostic - General: 320
Private General Room			Room and Board- Private 110
Order - Blood Examination	Microscopic examination of blood	ICD 9 - CM: 90.59	General Lab: 300

Syringe		HCPCS: A4657	Medical/Surgical Equipment 0278
Physician Charges			Professional Fees: 988 Consultation
Food Services			Patient Convenience: 991 Cafeteria/Guest Tray
Diphenoxylate 2.5 MG		RxNorm: 329305	General Drugs: 251

DAY 03	Description	Code	Revenue Code
Order - Blood Examination	Microscopic examination of blood	ICD 9 - CM: 90.59	General Lab: 300
Private General Room			Room and Board- Private 110
Syringe		HCPCS: A4657	Medical/Surgical Equipment 0278
Physician Charges			Professional Fees: 988 Consultation
Food Services			Patient Convenience: 991 Cafeteria/Guest Tray
Diphenoxylate 2.5 MG		RxNorm: 329305	General Drugs: 251

DAY 04	Description	Code	Revenue Code
Final Diagnosis	Food Poisoning	ICD 9 - 005.9	
Private General Room			Room and Board- Private 110
Food Services			Patient Convenience: 991 Cafeteria/Guest Tray
Physician Charges			Professional Fees: 988 Consultation
Diphenoxylate 2.5 MG		RxNorm: 329305	General Drugs: 251

As mentioned in our previous discussions, once the Patient is discharged, in this case, after four days, Medical Coding will happen. Some of the codes which the Medical Coder will code for are listed below. These include the procedure codes and Diagnosis Codes and the Final diagnosis code.

Medical Coding		
Primary Diagnosis	Food Poisoning	ICD 9 - 005.9
		Other Injury, Poisoning & Toxic Effect Diag W Mcc
Procedure Code	Order - X-Ray	CPT Code: 74010 - XR ABD COMPLETE

In parallel, the Billing system will also refer to something called the Charge Master, which contains the list of Charges defined by the hospital.

Charge Master			
Item	**Revenue Code**	**HCPCS Code**	**Standard Price**
Private General Room	Room and Board- Private 110		$200.00
Physician Charges	Professional Fees: 988 Consultation		$300.00
Food Services	Patient Convenience: 991 Cafeteria/Guest Tray		$100.00
Diphenoxylate 2.5 MG	General Drugs: 251		$20.00
Order - X-Ray	Radiology Diagnostic - General: 320		$400.00
Order - Blood Examination	General Lab: 300		$200.00
Syringe	Medical/Surgical Equipment 0278	A4657	$2.00

In this case, assuming we are using the % of Coverage method and below is a break-up for each charge line. Humana is the primary insurance for Mr. Brown while Cigna is the secondary insurance. One does not send the Insurance Claim to both Payers at once. At first, the Primary insurance company will receive the patient details insurance; after the primary processing, the secondary insurance company will receive the claim file.

	% Covered by Humana	% Covered by Cigna
Private General Room	30	0
Physician Charges	40	30
Food Services	80	0
Diphenoxylate 2.5 MG	60	0
Order - X-Ray	70	10
Order - Blood Examination	50	30
Syringe	0	0

This process is Co-ordination of benefits, in which Multiple payers work together to get most of the coverage for the Patient.

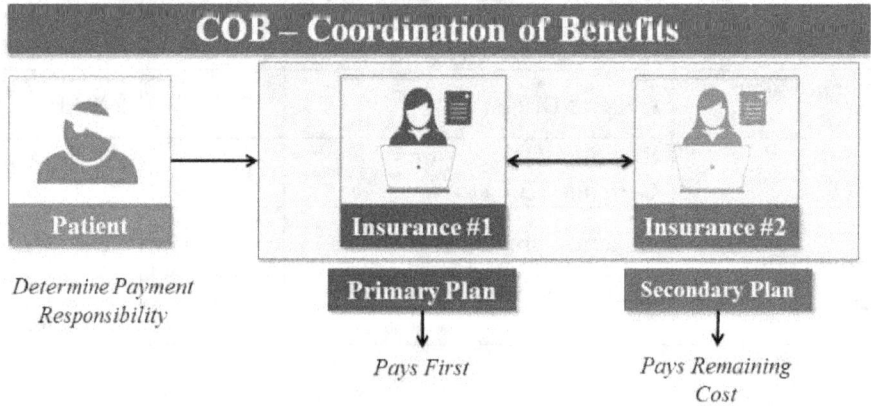

Figure: Co-Ordination of Benefits

In the case of Mr. Brown, we can calculate the total charges by multiplying the quantity, as shown below.

Item	Quantity	Charges	Total
Private General Room	4 (days)	$200	$800
Physician Charges	4 (days)	$300	$1,200
Food Services	4 (days)	$100	$400
Diphenoxylate 2.5 MG	4	$20	$80
Order - X-Ray	1	$400	$400
Order - Blood Examination	2 times	$200	$400
Syringe	2	$2	$4
			$3,284

Now from this total amount, we calculate how much will be paid by Humana and how much by Cigna.

Item	Humana		Cigna	
	% Covered	$ Amount	% Covered	$ Amount
Private General Room	30	$240	0	$0
Physician Charges	40	$480	30	$360
Food Services	80	$320	0	$0
Diphenoxylate 2.5 MG	60	$48	0	$0
Order - X-Ray	70	$280	10	$40
Order - Blood Examination	50	$200	30	$120
Syringe	0	$0	0	$0
		$1,568		$520

Finally, we have calculated what each Insurance company will pay and what the Patient will have to pay at the end, which is $1,196/-. The amount calculated is known as Co-Insurance in Medical Billing Terminology.

	Total Charges	Humana Payment	Payment by Cigna	Co-Insurance (Patient Pays)
Private General Room	$800.00	$240.00	$0.00	$560.00
Physician Charges	$1,200.00	$480.00	$360.00	$360.00
Food Services	$400.00	$320.00	$0.00	$80.00
Diphenoxylate 2.5 MG	$80.00	$48.00	$0.00	$32.00
Order - X-Ray	$400.00	$280.00	$40.00	$80.00
Order - Blood Examination	$400.00	$200.00	$120.00	$80.00
Syringe	$4.00	$0.00	$0.00	$4.00
	$3,284.00	$1,568.00	$520.00	$1,196.00

Please note, this is a hypothetical example, and this is a very basic way of calculating the coverage and other details. In actual, the process is very complicated with multiple rules which need to be considered. This example was added so that one could get some basic understanding of how the calculation is done.

#16 My List of Codes

Till now, you would have realized there are many terminologies in Healthcare and very difficult to remember each. If you want to understand each, then HL7 (Value Codes) might be where you start as it captures every possible information /event which can happen in healthcare. But if you are looking for a summary of some of the codes, the table below should give a good start.

Sr. No.	Term	Description	Usage
01.	ICD 9	International Classification of Diseases the 9th version	Diagnosis Codes & Procedures
02.	ICD 10	International Classification of Diseases the 10th version	Diagnosis Codes & Procedures
03.	SNOMED -CT	Systematized Nomenclature of Medicine -- Clinical Terms	Clinical Terminology
04.	RxNorm	Normalized names for clinical drugs	Drug Codes
05.	NDC	National Drug Code used for each medication	Drug Codes
06.	NDFRT	The National Drug File - Reference Terminology	Drug Codes
07.	LOINC	Logical Observation Identifiers Names and Codes	Lab Results/Observations
08.	CVX	Vaccine administered code set	Immunization Codes
09.	MVX	Manufacturers of Vaccines	Manufacturing Codes
10.	Type of Bill	Four Digit Code used on the UB04 form	UB04 Claim file
11.	Condition Codes	Code used on the claim file which can affect payer processing	UB04 Claim file

		e.g. 22 = Patient on Multiple drug Regime	
12.	Occurrence Code	These are codes related to a specific date, e.g., 01 = Auto Accident - date of the accident	UB04 Claim file
13.	Value Code	Indicates the type of Service, payment or coverage e.g. A0 = Ambulance service present on claim	UB04 Claim file
14.	Revenue Code	Indicates where the patient was provided treatment in the hospital e.g. 0123 = Pediatric	UB04 Claim file
15.	HCPCS Code	They are also called as Level 2 CPT codes used to code 1. Services 2. Supplies 3. Materials 4. Procedures	UB04 Claim file
16.	NPI	National Provider Index - Unique 10-digit identifier assigned to Healthcare Providers by CMS	UB04 Claim file
17.	CPT Codes	These are called as Level 1 CPT Codes; they are used to describe surgeries, tests, evaluations	UB04 Claim file
18.	Coding Modifier	Indicates alteration to a service or procedure performed e.g., Modifier 22- Increased Medical Services	UB04 Claim file
19.	DRG	Diagnosis Related Grouping (There are Grouper Software's)	Billing Calculation
20.	MDC	Major Diagnostic Categories - Formed by dividing all principle diagnosis codes into 25 mutually exclusive areas	Billing Calculation

#17 References

1 Million+ Stunning Free Images to Use Anywhere - Pixabay, pixabay.com.

"2015 ICD-9-CM Procedure 14. * : Operations On Retina, Choroid, Vitreous, And Posterior Chamber." *The Web's Free ICD-9-CM & ICD-10-CM Medical Coding Reference*, www.icd9data.com/2015/Volume3/08-16/14/default.htm.

"45 CFR § 164.526 - Amendment of Protected Health Information." *LII / Legal Information Institute*, www.law.cornell.edu/cfr/text/45/164.526.

American Public Health Association (APHA) Publications, ajph.aphapublications.org/.

Centers for Disease Control and Prevention, 21 May 2019, www.cdc.gov/.

CNBC, 21 May 2019, www.cnbc.com.

"Diabetes: Medical Attention for Nephropathy." *ECQI Resource Center | The One-stop Shop for the Most Current Resources to Support Electronic Clinical Quality Improvement*, 16 May 2019, ecqi.healthit.gov/ecqm/measures/cms134v5.

"DICOM, Digital Imaging and Communications in Medicine." *SIIM.org*, siim.org/page/DICOM.

Federal Register, www.federalregister.gov/.

Flickr, www.flickr.com/.

Free Stock Photos · Pexels, www.pexels.com/.

Gartner, www.gartner.com.

HealthITAnalytics. *Healthcare IT Analytics News on Healthcare BI, Population Health and Data Management - HealthITAnalytics*, healthitanalytics.com/.

Holland & Hart Health Law Blog, www.hhhealthlawblog.com/.

Home - Centers for Medicare & Medicaid Services, 21 May 2019,
www.cms.gov/.

"ICD-10 Codes." *MicroMD*, www.micromd.com/icd-10/icd-10-codes/.

"Individuals? Right Under HIPAA to Access Their Health Information."
HHS.gov, 25 Feb. 2016, www.hhs.gov/hipaa/for-
professionals/privacy/guidance/access/index.html.

"Jacques Bertillon (1851-1922)." *MacTutor History of Mathematics*, www-
history.mcs.st-andrews.ac.uk/Biographies/Bertillon.html.

*LOINC — The Freely Available Standard for Identifying Health Measurements,
Observations, and Documents*, loinc.org/.

"MDC 03 - Diseases & Disorders of the Ear, Nose, Mouth & Throat." *ICD-10
Code Lookup*, icd10coded.com/ms-drg/mdc-03/.

National Center for Biotechnology Information, www.ncbi.nlm.nih.gov/.

Noun Project, thenounproject.com/.

"Nuance - PDF, Customer Service, HIM, and Speech Recognition Solutions."
Nuance Communications, www.nuance.com/index.html.

*Ophthalmology EMR | Charity, Trust, Mission Hospital ERP, GST, NABH | EMR
Software | Indoor Positioning Systems*, 3 Mar. 2019,
www.hospitalinformationsystem.com/.

PokitDok, pokitdok.com/.

"Respiratory Therapies." *Fitzsimmons Home Medical Equipment*,
www.fitzhme.com/conditions-and-therapies/respiratory-therapies/.

"What is DICOM (Digital Imaging and Communications in Medicine)? -
Definition from WhatIs.com." *SearchHealthIT*,
searchhealthit.techtarget.com/definition/DICOM-Digital-Imaging-and-
Communications-in-Medicine.

Black, Caroline. "Hanks, Barrymore, Schwarzenegger: Medical Files Breached
at UCLA, Researcher Convicted." *Live, Breaking News Today: Latest
National Headlines, World News and More from CBSNews.com and
Watch the CBSN Live News Stream 24x7*, 29 Apr. 2010,

www.cbsnews.com/news/hanks-barrymore-schwarzenegger-medical-
files-breached-at-ucla-reseacher-convicted/

"Data Sharing Practices of Medicines Related Apps and the Mobile Ecosystem:
Traffic, Content, and Network Analysis." *The BMJ*, 20 Mar. 2019,
www.bmj.com/content/364/bmj.l920.

"Failure to Terminate Former Employee's PHI Access Costs Colorado Hospital
$111,400." *HIPAA Journal*, 12 Dec. 2018,
www.hipaajournal.com/failure-to-terminate-former-employees-phi-
access-costs-colorado-hospital-111400/.

"FindLaw's United States Ninth Circuit Case and Opinions." *Findlaw*,
caselaw.findlaw.com/us-9th-circuit/1600563.html

"First Lawsuit Against Facebook over Cambridge Analytica Filed in
Washington, D.C." *NBC News*, 19 Dec. 2018,
www.nbcnews.com/tech/tech-news/first-lawsuit-against-facebook-over-
cambridge-analytica-filed-washington-d-n949956.

"Germ Theory." *Science Museum*,
broughttolife.sciencemuseum.org.uk/broughttolife/techniques/germtheor
y.

Harish C. Rijhwani. "Internet of Things? A Myth or Reality for Healthcare: IoT
or Internet of Things Has Been Around for Quite a Long Time Now, It
Was in 1999 when Kevin Ashton Coined the Term Internet of
Things." *Becker's Hospital Review*,
www.beckershospitalreview.com/healthcare-information-
technology/internet-of-things-a-myth-or-reality-for-healthcare.html.

HealthITSecurity. "Majority of Health Apps Share User Data, Without
Transparency." *HealthITSecurity*, 21 Mar. 2019,
healthitsecurity.com/news/majority-of-health-apps-share-user-data-
without-transparency.

"HIPAA Violation Cases." *HIPAA Journal*, 30 Nov. 2017,
www.hipaajournal.com/hipaa-violation-cases/.

Rijhwani, Harish. "Healthcare Decoded - History of Medical
       Records." *LinkedIn*, www.linkedin.com/pulse/healthcare-decoded-
       history-medical-records-harish-rijhwani/.

---. "Healthcare Decoded - The Ice Breaker." *LinkedIn*,
       www.linkedin.com/pulse/healthcare-decoded-ice-breaker-harish-
       rijhwani/.

---. "Healthcare Decoded- The Rise of Health Insurance." *LinkedIn*,
       www.linkedin.com/pulse/healthcare-decoded-rise-health-insurance-
       harish-rijhwani/.

---. "Untitled - Preface." *LinkedIn*, www.linkedin.com/pulse/untitled-preface-
       harish-rijhwani/.

"Telemedicine - The 100 Year Old Prediction." *LinkedIn*,
       www.linkedin.com/pulse/telemedicine-100-year-old-prediction-harish-
       rijhwani/.

Using Evidence to Improve Population Health | Milbank Memorial Fund,
       www.milbank.org/wp-content/uploads/2016/10/DONABEDIAN-2005-
       The_Milbank_Quarterly.pdf.

Pixabay.com. (2019). Free Image on Pixabay - X-Ray, Equipment. [online]
       Available at: https://pixabay.com/photos/x-ray-equipment-666919/.

Dicomstandard.org. (2019). History – DICOM Standard. [online] Available at:
       https://www.dicomstandard.org/history/.

#18 Glossary of Terms

www.ingramcontent.com/pod-product-compliance
Lightning Source LLC
Chambersburg PA
CBHW081001170526

45158CB00010B/2870